You Are Not Alone

An anthology of perinatal mental health stories
from conception to postpartum

You Are Not Alone

An anthology of perinatal mental health stories
from conception to postpartum

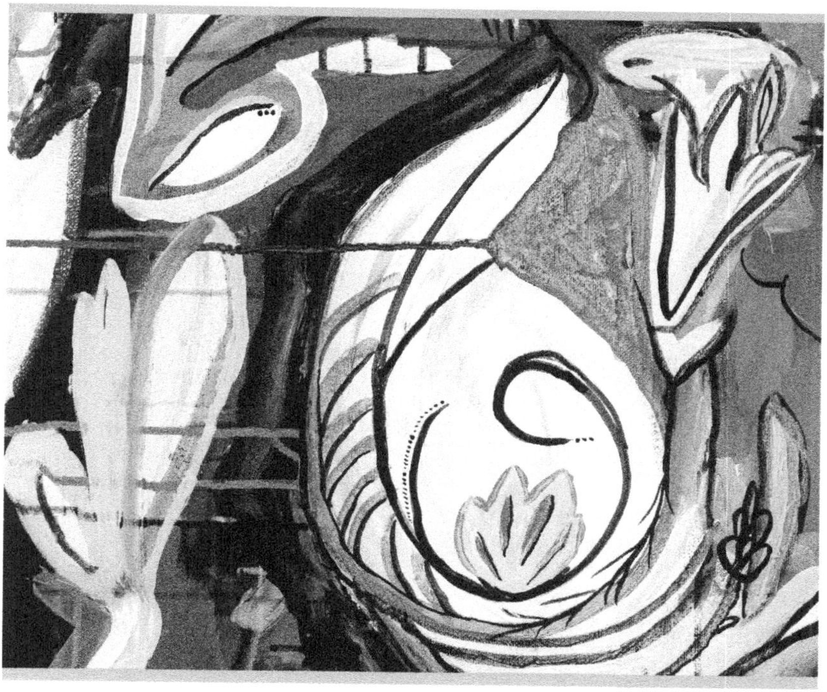

Special chapter on anxiety & intrusive thoughts by Karen Kleinman
plus insights from top perinatal mental health experts

CANADIAN PERINATAL MENTAL HEALTH COLLABORATION

echo BOOKS

Wintertickle PRESS

Wintertickle Press
132 Commerce Park Drive,
Unit K, Ste. 155
Barrie, ON
L4N 0Z7

Winterticklepress.bom
FB/WintertickIePress

ISBN 9781989664087

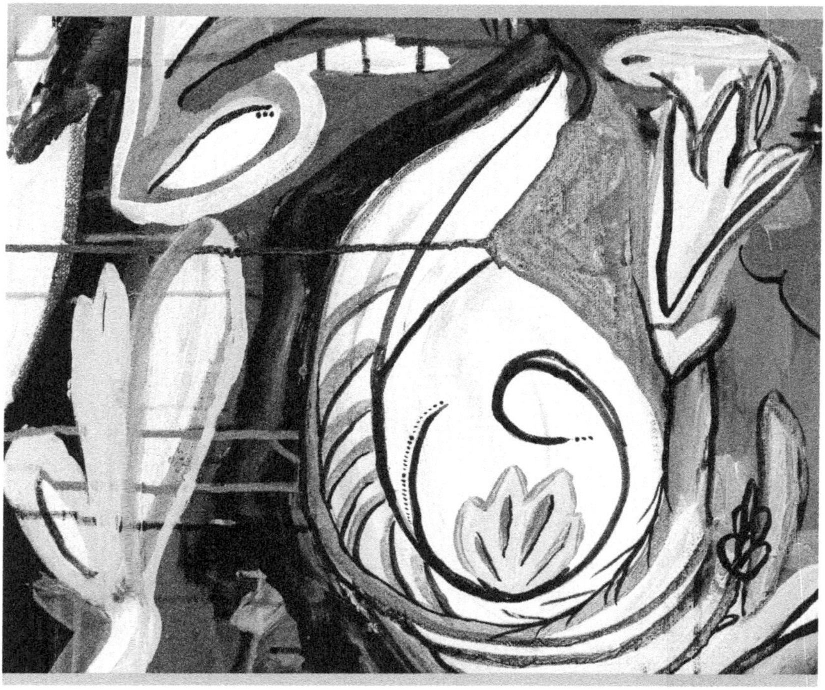

Cover art by Kayla Huszar, Regina, Saskatchewan

FLOW

This painting is the beauty that is in every mother.

The beauty that is in every child.

The sacrifice.

The grief.

The identity.

The shifts.

The same.

Everything has its own place.

The story of motherhood can be dark, light, swirly, jagged, all of it at the same time.

Who are we?

Mother. Human. Emotion.

Beauty. Pain. Tense.

Grounded. Resilient.

All of it. All of me. All of you.

FLOW

Kayla Huszar, BSW, RSW, is a maternal mental health specialist. She advocates for self-care. She has this special way of erasing your mom-guilt. Nature, coffee, pastels, and intuitive painting are her favorite things, besides her fur and human kids. She is also a self-proclaimed, recovering perfectionist mama, who eats a lot of Oreos. Kayla supports women through pregnancy, postpartum, and motherhood through 1:1, groups and workshops rooted in body-centred expressive art therapy. Connect with Kayla on Instagram @kayla.huszar

A word after a word after a word is power.

~ Margaret Atwood

CONTENT & TRIGGER WARNING

The contents of this book will include discussion and description of perinatal mental illness experiences that may be difficult and/or triggering for some. Some topics may include, but are not limited to, prenatal and postpartum depression, anxiety, obsessive-compulsive disorder, post-traumatic stress disorder, bipolar disorder, psychosis, miscarriage, stillbirth, and suicidal ideation.

DISCLAIMER

The information in this book is not meant to provide medical advice for individuals. Anyone seeking medical help should consult their primary health-care provider or seek assistance at their nearest hospital emergency department. For a list of perinatal mental health care practitioners in your area, please visit Postpartum Support International at www.postpartum.net or call/text 1-800-944-4773.

TABLE OF CONTENTS

FOREWORD

A BEAUTIFUL, YOUNG, SUCCESSFUL WOMAN who had become psychotic very shortly after giving birth to her first baby used to do public talks with me about perinatal mental health. She had become so sick by two weeks postpartum that she required intensive inpatient psychiatric care.

One day, while driving her home after we had talked to a group of mothers, she asked me why prenatal classes didn't teach about postpartum depression or psychosis. I said, they do. There is a one-hour session just about anxiety, and depression and they introduce the local support group held in the same building. She was surprised.

She and her husband had attended these prenatal classes, but she didn't remember this at all. We chatted about it, and we realized that because they were so happy to be pregnant, she and her husband never thought it would affect her and never thought that she would become depressed. So they didn't pay much attention during the session, instead focusing on breastfeeding and bathing the baby, which they did worry about.

She didn't remember feeling depressed, and she was unaware of her behaviour. She was treated properly in the psychiatric unit and gained confidence in her mothering through the support of the postpartum depression support group. She went on to have two physically and mentally healthy pregnancies and lovely babies. All of the family continues to thrive, but had she not gotten quick and appropriate treatment, it could have turned out quite differently as it sadly does for many other people.

You Are Not Alone is an anthology that highlights mother's and people's experiences with maternal and perinatal mood disorders that teaches us about their pain, confusion, and guilt during this time of expected joy. Reading these heart-wrenching stories, I was struck by some of the comments and how central they are to people who struggle with perinatal mood problems, yet how universally unexpected they are by new mothers and their families. These words, as their stories, illustrate these similarities.

On expectations and reality:

"I realized that she could sleep in the same thing she wore during the day and nobody would notice."

"I'm not experiencing motherhood the way I thought I would."

"I should be able to do it on my own."

On being nurtured:

"Looking back, I believe a period of rest and nurturing would have led to a much different experience of early motherhood for me."

"There is no tribe around us."

"Without the option to sleep or take a break from my responsibilities, the threat of death seems more real today."

People continue to die or have permanently altered lives and relationships as a result of unidentified or undertreated perinatal mood disorders. We must start by dispelling the fairytale dreams of idyllic motherhood and get people the support they need once and for all.

Whilst there is anxiety and despair in their stories, there is also hope that they can help others see that they are not alone, that mothers can and do survive. This necessary collection puts a face to this advocacy movement to increase awareness and get public policy and support for our mothers and their children, our next generation.

Dr. Angela Bowen is Professor Emeritus at the University of Saskatchewan. She is a Registered Nurse and trained midwife. Angela is the author of 50 articles, as well as *MotherFirst: Maternal Mental Health Strategy in Saskatchewan*, and *Today's Grandmother: Your Guide to the First Two Years*. She was co-lead on the Registered Nurses Association of Ontario Best Practices for Perinatal Depression. Angela founded Maternal Mental Health Day in Saskatchewan, which has become a global event. Her research has included CIHR and other funding to develop and evaluate the Maternal Mental Health Program that she spearheaded in Saskatoon, longitudinal studies of antenatal depression to five years postpartum, knowledge translation and policy development for maternal mental health, and Indigenous maternal wellness.

INTRODUCTION

THIS BOOK IS TRULY A dream come true.

We have to admit, however, that putting together this anthology during a pandemic amid a lockdown with kids and dishes and deadlines was super hard, but we knew we had to push through and do it anyway.

We just couldn't sit on these stories.

We knew we needed to get them out as quickly as we could because as much as we were going nuts being stuck at home with so much on our plates, we also knew rates of perinatal mental illness were soaring way above what they were pre-pandemic.

We knew moms and dads and partners and people needed support now, more than at any other time in recent history. So we leaned in and let the laundry pile up. We yelled at our husbands to pitch in even more, said eff-it to the pile of mismatched socks, and fervently got to work. And even if COVID-19 suddenly vanished by the time we published and life went back to normal, we knew many would still need support to recover from the trauma of having lived through an unpredictable and life-altering pandemic.

This anthology is about more than postpartum depression as our title suggests. It's about preconception and pregnancy too. This book contains stories that span the spectrum of perinatal mental illness including infertility, miscarriage, disability, tokophobia, stillbirth, prenatal and postpartum anxiety, obsessive-compulsive disorder, bipolar disorder, and psychosis along with what it's like to struggle with a perinatal mental illness during an unprecedented global pandemic.

This anthology features stories primarily by cisgender women and the words mom and mother are prominent throughout. Many of the experiences shared in this anthology likely resonate with people of all sexual and gender identities. However, it is vital that in our efforts to improve perinatal mental health across Canada, that we be inclusive with regard to sexual and gender identity—as well as to other identities and groups who experience marginalization and oppression, such as people with disabilities and Black, Indigenous, People of Colour (BIPOC).

Like sexual and gender minority populations, these groups often experience discrimination and mistreatment in the perinatal period as well as high rates of adverse perinatal health outcomes, including adverse perinatal mental health outcomes.

When we put the call out for stories, we were overwhelmed with the response. We could fill volumes with the amount of submissions we received, which speaks to the willingness of people who want to share their experiences and support others. It also confirms that we have a national crisis on our hands.

The idea for a perinatal mental health anthology first came to us after we met in 2015. Patricia was a journalist for *HuffPost Canada*, blogging about her perinatal mental health journey as well as writing articles about the state of perinatal mental health in Canada. She interviewed experts across the country including Jaime, an advanced practice nurse/psychotherapist and Ontario's first and only regional perinatal mental health coordinator.

During our interview, we talked about our own experiences and how 20% of women and 10% of men in Canada develop postpartum depression and how we believe that number to be much higher. We discussed how Canada is lagging behind other countries in providing universal screening and timely access to treatment. We talked about how, of those who come forward asking for help, only 15% receive it. We talked about how damaging the effects of untreated perinatal mental illness are on the mother, birthing person, father, partner, family, and on children who grow up to be more at risk of developing a mental illness, as well as society, the economy, and the very health and wellbeing of our future generation.

We talked a lot.

Our friendship was immediate and pretty convenient since we learned we only lived a few couple kilometres apart from one another in the city of Barrie. We started bumping into each other at the grocery store and meeting up in coffee shops frustrated there wasn't an organized effort in Canada to advocate for better perinatal care.

It wasn't long before we decided that we needed to stop talking in aisle six and start taking action. So one day, we took a leap of faith, jumped in head and heart first, and co-founded Canada's first perinatal mental health advocacy group, the Canadian Perinatal Mental Health Collaborative, or CPMHC for short.

Many thought we were crazy and at times we did, too. Here we were, two extremely busy moms with full time jobs and no funding, forging ahead on a wing and prayer with an unrelenting passion to change the system. One cold snowy night at one of our favourite local java haunts, we spent hours brainstorming our vision and jotting down all our ideas, and we just went for it. We got our social media profiles up and running and started running campaigns. We weren't afraid to put ourselves out there and make mistakes because we were committed to our mission and to learning.

We officially launched in 2019, and our first campaign was a call we put out to everyone who shared our passion to come join us in our efforts. And you definitely heard us! In no time, we were able to assemble a team of researchers and clinicians to form a national committee with representation from each province and territory. We gathered an equally impressive team of savvy social media ambassadors, all with as much passion and determination as we had in order to lobby the government for a national perinatal mental health strategy.

During the federal election, we reached out to each party leader and were ecstatic to receive a personal letter of support from NDP leader Jagmeet Singh. In the wings were whispers of support from the other parties as well, including the Liberal party, which went on to form the government. This was an all-party affair, and we were vying to get everyone on board. We strived to make as much noise as we could. The media thought we had an important story to tell. We quickly became known as the two "Barrie moms on a mission" to improve perinatal mental health care in Canada. Our little engine that could was suddenly on the map, and we were being taken seriously by the perinatal mental health community. Perhaps our dream would be realized sooner than what we could have ever thought possible.

And then the pandemic hit.

Schools and businesses closed, and it seemed like everything was suddenly put on hold. We wondered whether we should stop, too. Weeks turned into months, and we all soon realized that this pandemic wasn't going anywhere anytime soon. In fact, our call for a national strategy was becoming even more crucial.

Women and birthing persons grappled with not having their partners and support persons present with them during birth. New parents were not able to draw on the support from family and friends postpartum, many while trying to juggle caring for a newborn and children who were unexpectedly home all day because of school and daycare closures. Many parents also feared they would contract COVID-19 and pass it along to their infants.

So we forged on.

On World Maternal Mental Health Day, an international annual awareness campaign that falls on the first Wednesday each May, we launched our biggest social media campaign to date. We asked people to send us a video of themselves telling us why Canada needed a national perinatal mental health strategy #NowMoreThanEver. For a month leading up to World Maternal Mental Health Day, we shared videos from people with lived experience, mayors, provincial and federal ministers, and celebrities who fearlessly supported our campaign including actors Juno Rinaldi and Sarah McVie from *Workin' Moms*, and comedian and author, Jessica Holmes.

We also launched a petition that was presented virtually to the House of Commons by federal MP Heather McPherson of Edmonton-Strathcona who has become one of Canada's first political and vocal perinatal mental health champions along with Ontario Parkdale-High Park MPP Bhutila Karpoche whom we are working with and supporting in her efforts to legislate improved maternal mental health care in Ontario.

After receiving a lacklustre response to our petition from the federal government, (or as one of our national committee members aptly described as a "dog's breakfast" of piecemeal programs that don't adequately address perinatal mental health), we pushed ahead and delivered our very first report to the government on May 5, 2021, containing our recommendations for a national strategy.

Our report also contained results from a first-ever national survey for health-care practitioners that we conducted with the University of

Calgary. Our data showed that the majority of health-care practitioners surveyed did not receive specialized training in perinatal mental health and that some patients languish on wait lists for up to 12 months before getting the help they so desperately need.

On May 5, 2021, MP McPherson delivered our Motion to the House of Commons calling for all MPs to recognize World Maternal Mental Health Day in Canada and to support the idea of creating a national perinatal mental health strategy. The Motion carried unanimously and on June 3, 2021, history was made once again with the introduction and passing of first reading of Private Member's Bill C-306 brough forward by MP Don Davies calling for a National Perinatal Mental Health Strategy Act.

We just want people in Canada to have what people in the U.K., Australia, and parts of the U.S. already have—universal screening and timely access to the best evidence-based treatment for the most common complication of pregnancy and postpartum.

We also set about creating this anthology filled with 49 stories for people across the 49th parallel—and beyond. Perinatal mental illness knows no boundaries. Each author bravely tells their story of their own lived experience in their own words and many of them have gone on to become fierce advocates themselves.

In addition to the personal stories, there are chapters written by top perinatal mental health experts who were more than happy to contribute their knowledge, expertise, and advice.

We are so thankful to have widely renowned perinatal mental health advocates Karen Kleiman and Dr. Nichole Fairbrother collaborate on a chapter about postpartum anxiety and intrusive thoughts. We are also thrilled to have chapters written for us by many more incredible health-care professionals including: Dr. Simone Vigod, Dr. Ariel Dalfen, Dr. Ryan Van Lieshout, Dr. Verinder Sharma, Dr. Anja Wittkowski, Dr. Gail Erlick Robertson, Dr. Jodi Pawluski, Dr. Lesley Tarasoff, Dr. Christine Ou, and Mark Williams, founder of International Fathers Mental Health Day and the #HowAreYouDad campaign.

We hope these stories help you realize that you are not alone and that there is a growing movement of advocates dedicated to bringing about change.

One day, we hope you'll join us.

Patricia Tomasi & Jaime Charlebois
Co-Founders, www.cpmhc.ca
Facebook: Canadian Perinatal Mental Health Collaborative
Instagram: @cpmhc
Twitter: @canpmhc

Part 1:

Preconception,
Pregnancy
&
Birth

my body

my mind
even my taste buds have changed
my perception on life
my ability to love

everything

and you are not even here yet

Tyneisha Ternent, Bearing Fruit
@tythepoetess

TOKOPHOBIA

Aline St-Denis

I GOT MY PERIOD AT age 12.

Mom tries her best to explain what is happening to me, but all I feel is a confused mix of emotions. I feel proud that I am becoming a woman, sure, but I also feel incredibly anxious about what I perceive to be the *danger* of becoming pregnant.

I feel helpless and a sense of injustice with this new function of my body. I also find it uncomfortable and embarrassing. It seems to me that it is much easier for boys who have none of this to worry about. And why is it so painful if it's a natural process?

Mom's biggest fear is that I'll have two *illegitimate* pregnancies and an abortion like she did before getting *properly* married and having my brother and me. Mom suffers from generalized anxiety disorder and chronic depression.

Her way of protecting me from the horrors of childbirth is by instilling in me a terrifying fear of pregnancy and labour. From a young age, she tells me horrible stories. It doesn't help that a neighbour of ours dies in childbirth and one of my primary school teachers becomes paraplegic from a botched epidural.

I leave home at age 17.

I leave our small town to start working in the big city. I had just finished a secretary course, and leaving for a new job became the easiest and quickest way for me to get out of the toxic environment I was living in at home.

I experienced my first panic attack at age 19.

While watching a documentary about childbirth on television, suddenly, I became nauseous and everything went black. I started trembling and feeling very hot, like I was going to pass out. I didn't understand what was happening to me. Was it related to the images I was seeing on TV?

I am so terrified of becoming pregnant that at age 23, I ask my doctor if it's possible to become permanently sterilized. The gynecologist explains that it's not usual practice for a young, healthy woman such as me to request and have a tubal ligation procedure. He doesn't ask me why I want this intervention and I decide, in the end, not to do it.

I don't realize I'm suffering from tokophobia until age 55.

Tokophobia is the intense fear and anxiety of pregnancy and childbirth. I finally realized decades later that tokophobia is what I'd been suffering and still am suffering with today.

I also learn that I'm not the only one. Tokophobia is a crippling phobia that sneaks into my everyday life. Spoken or written words, pictures and any situation involving the subject of pregnancy or childbirth creates a lot of discomfort for me that manifests in panic attacks and fainting.

Cognitive behavioral therapy, eye movement integration, and medication have all provided me great benefits so that I can regain a balanced life. But I had to find all this out for myself and find therapists to help me.

Most tokophobic women want more than anything to start a family. So how can they get the help they need before they get pregnant? It is essential that women and persons have access to adequate treatment, regardless of whether they want to have children or not. Left untreated, tokophobia has the potential to seriously hinder a lifetime.

I would know.

Aline St-Denis has made it her mission to raise awareness about tokophobia. She voluntarily collaborates as a patient partner with a specialist in reproductive psychiatry and a clinical psychologist. You can find Aline on Twitter @Tocophobie

FEAR OF CHILDBIRTH

Dr. Nichole Fairbrother

I HAD REALLY BEAUTIFUL CHILDBIRTH experiences, but I knew of a lot of women who were really afraid of it. A lot of women I knew weren't sure they wanted to have children because they found childbirth so frightening. It just seemed really sad to me that a woman or person's fear could make it impossible to look forward to and experience the more beautiful parts of childbirth.

For some women, fear of childbirth or tokophobia (a phobia of childbirth) is so intense, it might lead them to an avoidance of pregnancy, even among women who really want to have children.

Although the prevalence of fear of childbirth has yet to be established, as many as 20 to 30% of women may be affected. In one study, fear of birth, in which symptoms met criteria for specific phobia was found to affect 2.5% of women who had never born a child and 4.5% of pregnant women who had two or more pregnancies.

Most women with a fear of childbirth suffer in silence. That's because there's little public awareness of fear of childbirth, and no standardized pathways for identifying and treating women with childbirth fear in Canada.

Several factors have been found to be associated with higher levels of childbirth fear including younger age, low social support, and dissatisfaction with a partner or support received from a partner. Mental health variables such as higher anxiety and stress, history of depression and depression during pregnancy, low confidence in one's ability to cope with labour and birth, and history of abuse have all been associated with higher levels of fear of childbirth.

In terms of physical health, higher levels of fatigue during pregnancy and lower self-rated health have also been associated with higher levels of fear of childbirth.

There is a strong association between previous negative birth experiences and/or traumatic births, and fear of childbirth. Studies have also shown that the odds of fear of childbirth increase with the number of obstetric complications experienced during a previous pregnancy. Women with a previous negative birth experience are five times more likely to experience fear of birth in a subsequent pregnancy.

History of prior operative or instrumental delivery has also been associated with higher levels of fear of childbirth. Although most studies have found a positive relationship between parity and fear of childbirth, with higher levels of childbirth fear reported by those who have never given birth (nulliparous) compared with those who have given birth to more than one child (multiparous), there is some evidence that the most severe levels of fear of childbirth are experienced by multiparous women.

Fear of birth specifically has been linked to more requests for epidural anesthesia during labour, longer labours and a higher likelihood of emergency and planned C-section. For instance, a study with 6,422 pregnant women from six European countries showed that 16.7% of women who had never born a child and 31.7% of pregnant women who had two or more pregnancies with severe fear of childbirth had a Cesarean section without medical indications (compared to 4.6% and 17.5% of women without severe fear of birth).

In one Finnish study, 8% of Cesarean sections at one hospital were potentially attributable to fear of vaginal delivery. Elevated fear of birth is consistently associated with preferences for C-sections among pregnant women and women who plan to become pregnant. There is also a higher likelihood of negative birth experiences among women with fear of childbirth, especially if the woman delivered by emergency C-section or instrumental vaginal delivery.

Historically, fear of childbirth has not been conceptualized as a diagnosable mental health condition, but rather a form of dimensional psychological distress characterized by fear and anxiety, and assessed via self-report inventory. This is problematic because, in the absence of clear diagnostic criteria, it may be difficult to determine the level at which the fear of childbirth may merit treatment.

All mood and anxiety and related conditions listed within the Diagnostic and Statistical Manual of Mental Disorders (DSM-5) require that symptoms of anxiety be either clinically distressing or life-interfering to the person experiencing them. Self-report measures typically assess distress only, but not life interference/impairment. To date, few if any studies have assessed self-report measures of fear of childbirth as screening tools for diagnosable anxiety conditions. In addition, it is not yet clear which of the various anxiety disorders may be the most appropriate fit for fear of childbirth. Specific phobia has been proposed as the most likely candidate, but this has yet to be tested. Specific phobias include fears of circumscribed objects and situations (e.g., fear of insects, animals, heights, blood, injections). Fear of childbirth is a circumscribed situation with symptoms and features closely resembling those of other specific phobias. Other possible candidates include health anxiety disorder and generalized anxiety disorder.

In collaboration with my colleagues at the University of British Columbia, we are developing a screening tool for childbirth fear: The Childbirth Fear Questionnaire (CFQ). We believe the CFQ will be an important step in identifying and treating women who suffer from severe prenatal fear of birth.

In addition to the most common fears of childbirth, which include labour pain and fear of harm to oneself or one's infant, the CFQ will be the first measure of fear of childbirth in which a fear of cesarean delivery is specifically assessed. We've also included subscales to assess fear of changes to one's body and sexual functioning, and fear of embarrassment during childbirth.

It's very normal to be a little fearful of childbirth, but for some women, their fear is at a level indicative of a diagnosable mental health condition. This implies that one's fear of childbirth is at a level of severity that is highly distressing or causing issues in that person's life.

In addition to the screening tool, we are also working on an online cognitive behaviour therapy program for pregnant women afraid of childbirth. Exposure-based CBT where women engage in gradual, controlled exposure to the source of their fear such as the fear of childbirth, gives women the opportunity to habituate or get used to that fear, so that their fear comes down. Exposure to childbirth can be in the form of stories, images, videos, and conversations.

Fear of childbirth is an important form of anxiety and distress for many pregnant people. Our lab is working to better identify and treat those who are experiencing this fear. Our hope is that our work will lead to better childbirth experiences for pregnant and birthing individuals.

Dr. Nichole Fairbrother is director of the Perinatal Anxiety Research Lab at the University of British Columbia. Dr. Fairbrother is a Clinical Associate Professor in the University of British Columbia's Department of Psychiatry, and a member of the Women's Health Research Institute at B.C. Women's Hospital. Dr. Fairbrother's research is in the area of reproductive mental health with a focus on new mothers' thoughts of infant-related harm and obsessive-compulsive disorder. More information about Dr. Fairbrother's work can be found on her web site at www.parlab.ubc.ca

WILL I BE ABLE?

Gabriella Carafa

IT'S TAKEN ME A LONG time to figure out how to start this story, a story not often told, but a story worth sharing. I ask myself questions like: *Does anybody even want to hear it? Will anyone feel comforted by these words?* But I still feel compelled to write it. I question whether my story even belongs in this book because unlike a lot of people who are a part of this book, I am not a parent. I am writing this story as a woman, a psychotherapist, and hopefully, one day, as a parent with a disability.

I was born with congenital hypotonia, a condition that means I have low muscle tone. There is no cure for it, and I have spent my entire life in a wheelchair. Being a parent has been one of the very few consistent goals in my life. It has never wavered. It has always been there. Sometimes it is as quiet as a whisper, and sometimes this wish is so loud I think everyone can hear it.

Growing up with a visible disability, parenting seemed so impossible when I thought of it in practical terms. When I think of my own mother, there are so many things that she provided for me and did for me growing up that I would not be physically able to do if I had my own child. But there were also other things that she did do, combined with the person that she is, that makes me feel that I would have a lot to offer a child.

Looking back at family photos and videos, you would be hard-pressed to find me without a doll or a real baby in my arms. I spent hours watching labour and delivery shows and could probably identify what Pitocin was by the age of seven. You see, I had a dream of being a parent, but I also had a dream of being part of the experience of people's pregnancy, labour and delivery, and the transition to parenthood.

As my disability is physical in nature, my dream of delivering babies was quickly put to the test. I would be asked: *How can you deliver babies with your fine motor skill challenges? Your wheelchair will be in the way. You won't be able to respond quickly enough if something goes wrong.* So I put the dream of working in the perinatal field to rest, and for a long time I believed I would never play a part in the perinatal world.

What I didn't put to rest, was my dream of one day becoming a mom.

I grew up in a very traditional Italian-Canadian family. I am the youngest, and both of my sisters have children. My eldest sister got married when I was six years old, and I asked her pretty much right away when she was going to have a baby.

My main goals when I was a child were to grow up, get married, and have a family. These goals were not imposed on me by my parents, in fact the opposite is true. They were trying to cope with having a disabled daughter and didn't know what life I could expect or hope for. Their main focus was to ensure that I pursued an education, got a job, and hopefully became a contributing member of society. My parents had a lot of fear that the world would not treat me the way my parents wanted me to be treated, and this impacted what they believed was possible for me. But still, my dream of getting married and having children was one that stayed with me.

As I was the only physically disabled person in my neighbourhood growing up, I did not have anyone who I could look up to. Regardless, I always believed that being a mom was possible for me. I just had to wait...wait until I got older, wait until I found a job, wait until I found the right person. Wait, wait, wait.

It wasn't until I entered my masters of social work program that I realized I could still be part of the perinatal working world, but maybe not in the way that I had expected. The moment I heard about perinatal social work, I knew it was for me. That was it. That was what I was meant to do. It combined something I loved with my abilities in a way I could be successful.

After I graduated, I worked in paediatric rehab for many years. What struck me working with parents was that they remembered the social worker that they had worked with when their child was first born or newly diagnosed. They remembered the support that they received, they remembered those conversations. When I transitioned into a perinatal social work role, my lived experience in combination with the experiences as a social worker that I acquired, gave me a different perspective.

Planning to have a baby, pregnancy, labour and delivery, and parenting are filled with so much hope and fear. We have so many hopes for that child, for ourselves, and for things to go according to plan. In reality, there are so many things that we cannot control or predict. I wanted to be that support person who was aware of all of the actual uncertainty in that period and who provided hope. I wanted to be the person who supported people when things did not go according to plan, when there was heartbreak, when there was loss.

My personal journey toward parenthood is still in progress. I am attempting to have a child on my own. I am so lucky that I now have friends with disabilities who have children. They have shown me it is possible. As I don't have a partner, I am alone on this journey to parenthood, a journey that has been bumpy so far, a journey that involves fertility appointments, uncertainty, and so many things that are not in my control.

I don't know what things will look like moving forward, but it is because of the amazing moms who I have worked with that I have the courage to keep going. They help me get through it with their stories of resilience, grief, heartbreak, and deep love. These moms are my hope, and I carry their stories with me on my own reproductive journey.

I may never be a parent. That dream might never come true for me, but I am grateful that I will always be a part of this world in some way, shape, or form. That dream has definitely come true.

Gabriella Carafa MSW RSW PMH-C is a social worker who is certified in perinatal mental health. She works as a perinatal social worker in acute care settings and as a transition strategy team lead in paediatric rehabilitation. Gabriella also has a private practice working with children, adolescents, adults, families and couples. Connect with Gabriella on Twitter @Gabriella_rsw

INFERTILITY

Lisa Tremayne

SEVENTY-TWO...

Seventy-two times I got my period and was so disappointed that my body had failed me.

Again.

Infertility.

I don't like how it feels.

But I am a maternal child health nurse, and I know where to go for help.

Seventy-two adds up to six years. Six years of infertility.

I am told I am of *advanced maternal age*. I am 34.

After one round of in vitro fertilization, I am lying on a gurney having my beautiful, large, round eggs extracted, 22 eggs to be exact. The eggs meet the sperm in a perfectly warm environment, and each day my husband and I receive updates as to how they are doing. Three days later, six zygotes are implanted back into my body.

Six.

The doctor is telling me not to get hopeful. One zygote is looking good, but the other five are being placed back inside my body to add to the possibility of that one embryo becoming a pregnancy. I lie on another gurney for an hour, willing that strong little group of cells to stick, to find a home inside me, and to fulfill my dream of becoming a mother.

Seven days later, in the hospital for ovarian hyper stimulation, I find out I am pregnant.

My body hasn't failed me this time.

We did it!

Then I'm told that there is a real possibility that I am pregnant...with twins.

Twins!

I am overjoyed.

We see two tiny little egg sacks. That's what they call them, egg sacks.

Two weeks later, I'm vomiting every day, all day, and we see another egg sack.

There. Are. Triplets. Inside. Of. Me.

Triplets!

I am somewhere between super impressed with my body and sheer terror. You see, as a nurse in this field, I know all the risks that come with *higher order multiples.* Four weeks after implantation, the doctor looks at me in utter disbelief. On the ultrasound screen, there are now *four* embryos.

I cry. I cry for me, I cry for these babies who are so desperately wanted, and I cry out for knowing too much of what can happen. I also haven't stopped vomiting in over a week. I am officially diagnosed with hyperemesis gravidarum and require hospitalization for dehydration.

Sometime between week 12 and 14, I lose one of my babies. At 30 weeks, I am diagnosed with pancreatitis and have been in labour five times, which had to be stopped with medication. I have been in the hospital all this time, and I am done. I want them out. I have nothing left to give. I am a shell of the person I was just seven-and-a-half weeks ago. I want to be a mom, yes, but I felt like a host, like I was being kept pregnant to grow these babies as big and strong as my body will allow. And that's it.

A short time later, I deliver two baby boys and one baby girl. One of my sons is born not breathing, and the other two are so tiny, barely over two pounds each. They are all whisked away after the briefest of glimpses, my tiny angels whom I completely adore.

Time gets fuzzy now. I remember being taken to the neonatal intensive care unit on the stretcher to see my babies. I am overwhelmed with emotion. My son is on a ventilator to assist his breathing and our other two babies are in incubators. They look fuzzy, yellow, and have lots of IVs.

The day is a blur. I feel like there is something wrong with me. I can't think properly and my heart feels like it's constantly racing. I'm cold. I am transferred to the intensive care unit in kidney failure and with too much fluid around my heart. Once again, I am alone, praying for my babies' birthday not to be the day they lose their mommy.

I don't remember the next five days in the ICU. I am brought out of my drug-induced haze on New Year's Eve and begin lying to get to my babies. *I am fine. I can get into a wheelchair. I can be moved to the step-down unit. Yes, yes, yes.* Whatever they needed me to say, I said it in order to be able to touch my babies.

I get to them. My heart explodes with love. I can feel my body wanting to lose consciousness from pushing it too far, too fast. I am able to will it away. I had heard of moms performing impossible feats for their children. This is my version as I will myself not to faint. I get to stay with my babies the rest of the day.

I am struck by my first *what if* thought. *What if I lose one of these babies? How will I survive?* My mom tells me not to worry, that they are in the best hands, in the best unit. She reminds me that I have always been a worrier.

I spend the next six weeks going back and forth from hospital to home, crying each time I have to leave without them. Finally, they all come home within five days of each other. Suddenly, I go from no babies to three babies. *I can handle it*, I tell myself. After all, I have been the nurse in charge of the nursery so often where at any given time there were 15 to 20 babies there.

I've got this.

There's no sleep to be had. I'm on a three-hour feeding schedule, with each feeding taking about two hours. I am completely undone. My worrying thoughts turn to non-stop racing thoughts. I am unable to sleep, even if all the babies are asleep at the same time. I feel rage building up inside me. I mention my racing thoughts to my obstetrician at my check-up, and he assures me that it's nothing and that I probably just need a shoe-shopping expedition to bring me back to normal.

I never mention what I'm feeling to him again or anyone else. I don't want others thinking I am unstable. I don't want my babies taken from me.

My feelings of anxiety and rage persist for months and months until I finally decide to tell my husband. He looks at me with disgust and says, "But you got everything you ever wanted."

I am a monster. I don't deserve these babies.

I start to become obsessed with death, about the many ways the babies could die. They could die in a house fire or by me driving my car off a bridge.

I start to avoid bridges.

I am suffering from severe untreated postpartum anxiety, obsessive-compulsive disorder, and intrusive thoughts. But I didn't know that to be the case until years later when working as a floor nurse on a postpartum unit, I recognized myself in the face of new mothers whom I know are feeling what I felt. That's when I decide I never want another mother to feel that way, to feel like a bad mom, to feel like a monster. I start sharing my phone number with moms, and I start getting them the help they need, therapy, and medication. These moms become my soul sisters.

New Jersey becomes the first state to mandate depression screenings for new moms before they leave the hospital. I am thrilled and fired up to do more. I start volunteering for a consortium that is getting these women the resources they need. I start an official postpartum depression support group and it quickly becomes the most attended support group at the hospital. My phone number keeps getting passed around from mom to mom with the message that *if you call or text this nurse, she will help you.*

I present an idea to my hospital for an actual postpartum depression program. There were none in the state—heck, there were only a handful in the whole country! It takes two years, but I finally get the go ahead and begin building the very program and services I know would have helped me.

The program quickly takes off. In less than two years, we officially become the Interdisciplinary Perinatal Mood and Anxiety Disorders Center at the Monmouth Medical Center in Long Branch with specialized treatment for new and expecting moms. I easily get over 50 new moms a month into the program. I tell each and every woman that this is the most common complication of childbirth, that one in five new moms will be hit with this illness, and most importantly, that perinatal mental illness is an actual illness.

Our peer-to-peer support group is the absolute crux of our center. The lived experience of a mom, who has been exactly where she is, feeling what she is feeling, thinking what she is thinking and sharing her journey with you is extremely healing.

I am thrilled to be part of a hospital system that understands the responsibility to take care of women's mental health as much as their physical health. I am blessed to be part of an amazing team of women, who are selfless and tireless in helping moms. This job has no clock. We are on, all the time.

By taking care of a new mom, we are taking care of her baby and her family. My calling is to keep moms healthy, in every way.

Lisa Tremayne is a registered nurse and mom of triplets plus one. Caroline was born just 20 months later. She works at the Monmouth Medical Center in Long Branch, New Jersey. In 2005, Lisa was involved in the development of New Jersey's universal mandatory screening program for prenatal and postpartum depression, the first of its kind in the U.S. In 2017, Lisa created and directed New Jersey's first Center for Perinatal Mood and Anxiety Disorders. Lisa also co-founded and acts as the president at the Bloom Foundation for Maternal Wellness. Connect with Lisa on Instagram @lisatremayne and @the_bloom_foundation_

PRENATAL MENTAL HEALTH

Dr. Gail Erlick Robinson

COMMON MYTH HAS IT THAT women during pregnancy are "blooming" and that postpartum is the most joyful time in women's lives. Unfortunately, this is not always true. Various factors preceding pregnancy as well as during pregnancy and postpartum can increase the risk of mental health problems during these times. It is important to recognize these risk factors, eliminate the ones that can be removed, and moderate the ones that cannot.

> *Ms. A is a 27-year-old married woman who is contemplating getting pregnant. There is a family history of depression in her mother and maternal aunt. Ms. A had depression at age 18, which responded to antidepressants and psychotherapy. She had a second depression at age 25 and is still taking an antidepressant. She has a very stressful job. She and her partner love each other, but they argue frequently. She came to discuss managing her pregnancy.*

Risk factors for depression or anxiety during pregnancy:

1. **History of mental health problems.** Women who have a personal or family history of depression, anxiety, or substance abuse have an increased vulnerability to developing mental health problems during pregnancy.
2. **Hormonal changes**. During pregnancy, there are dramatic changes in reproductive hormones. These are metabolically connected to chemicals in the brain responsible for maintaining mood. Many women find themselves more emotionally reactive during pregnancy. Women with a history of mental health problems are particularly vulnerable to these changes.

3. **Psychological pressures.** Even women who have chosen to become pregnant can have some doubts and concerns once the pregnancy is confirmed. With a firstborn, they now begin to anticipate how their life and freedom will change. The responsibility of becoming a parent may feel overwhelming. When adding to the family, the woman may have concerns about how she will manage with more than one child and what the impact will be on existing children.
4. **Stress related to the pregnancy.** Pregnancy can be a physically stressful time. Some women have severe cases of nausea and vomiting, which can last throughout the pregnancy. This interferes with their ability to gain weight and their general comfort level in life. If any kind of problem is detected with the pregnancy or with the baby, this will severely increase stress levels. Women, for example, who are found to have issues with their cervix and require cerclage (the placement of stitches to the cervix to hold it closed) or have to stay in bed due to bleeding during pregnancy will be under enormous stress, which can impact their mental health. If there are problems detected in the baby, women can remain anxious throughout the pregnancy. A previous history of miscarriage or infertility may also increase the risk of anxiety during pregnancy.

Other stressors:

Pregnant women are not immune to other life stressors. They may have concerns about finances or accommodation. They may struggle with job stress or unemployment. They may be coping with pre-existing physical illnesses that make it harder for them to handle the pregnancy or put them in a high risk category such as diabetes. All of these factors will add to the stress on the woman and make her more vulnerable to developing depression or an anxiety disorder.

Sexual abuse

Women who have been victims of sexual abuse might struggle with the examinations necessary during pregnancy and the delivery.

Social support

Good social support is a strong component of helping women stay well during pregnancy. Women benefit from having a good relationship with a partner, ongoing support from family and good friends. Women in dysfunctional or abusive relationships or who are distanced from their families are at added vulnerability. Those women who are on their own, do not have supportive families and feel isolated will have more difficulties coping with the pregnancy. They may already feel low and unhappy in their lives and the pregnancy may offset their loneliness or add to their distress.

Unwanted/unplanned pregnancies

An unwanted pregnancy may be an added risk factor for a woman's mental stability during pregnancy. How the woman comes to terms with this may depend on other stress factors in her life and whether she has good supports and a solid plan as to how she will manage when the baby is born. Many pregnancies are unplanned, but once over the surprise and perhaps shock of becoming pregnant, the woman is able to reconcile with being pregnant and start looking forward to the birth of the child.

Non-traditional pregnancies

Although the majority of pregnancies are in cis-gendered women, non-binary individuals and transgender men are also getting pregnant. The language and culture around pregnancy is highly gendered. Non-binary people may object to the use of female pronouns and language. Transgendered men might find it difficult to find care providers who are sensitive to their unique circumstances. They may feel stigmatized or ridiculed or have their gender identity denied.

All of these factors are cumulative. Those with a personal or family history of depression and who are also undergoing stresses specifically related to the pregnancy or external stressors with poor support systems, are at high risk of developing depression or anxiety during pregnancy.

Risk factors for bipolar disorder

Ms. B is a 30-year-old married teacher who is contemplating getting pregnant. She has a history of a first episode of depression at age 20. She was treated with antidepressants for nine months and then discontinued the medication. At age 26, she had a hypomanic episode and was treated with a mood stabilizer which she continued for six months. She has not been on any medication since that time. She has a family history of a paternal uncle who has bipolar disorder.

This case illustrates someone with a high risk of developing problems during pregnancy. Ms. B clearly has bipolar disorder. Bipolar disorders tend to be recurrent with episodes of depression and mania or hypermania, interspersed with times of mood stability. She has already had two episodes as well as having a family history of bipolar disorder. She has not been on any sustained medication and has been well for the last two years.

Individuals with bipolar disorder often struggle to adjust to the idea that they should be on sustained medication because they can have extended intervals of feeling well. Despite this, people with this disorder do better if they remain on a mood stabilizer, which can prevent them from developing depression or manic episodes. Depression during pregnancy can lead to severe distress and even suicidal ideation. A manic episode may cause the woman to act irrationally, use drugs or alcohol, or even develop delusional ideas or false beliefs about the pregnancy and the baby. This would, therefore, put her and the pregnancy at risk.

Risk factors for schizophrenia

Ms. C has a diagnosis of paranoid schizophrenia. She has had two episodes of illness during which she became very paranoid, was distrustful of others and heard voices talking to her. She was started on an antipsychotic medication but discontinued it after her first episode. Since her second episode three years ago, she has been maintained on this medication and has been well.

Schizophrenia is also a recurrent mental health disorder. This is a high-risk pregnancy as, without ongoing treatment, Ms. C runs the risk of having a recurrence during the pregnancy. At that time, she may develop false beliefs about the baby or the pregnancy and be at risk of harming herself or the baby.

Risk factors for other psychiatric disorders

There are other psychiatric disorders that may become more severe during pregnancy. Women with obsessive-compulsive disorders may have an increase of symptoms that cause them anxiety and distress including obsessive thoughts, compulsive hand washing, or cleaning and increased rituals such as constantly having to check and re-check. Women with a history of post-traumatic stress disorder may have an exacerbation of their symptoms of anxiety, nightmares, intrusive thoughts, and flashbacks as they contemplate a delivery and worry that something will go wrong during that time. Women with personality disorders that affect their sense of wellbeing, and relationships with others may feel overwhelmed by the demands of the pregnancy and the contemplation of becoming parents and having to look after a child.

Ms. A illustrates a number of risk factors. She has a personal and family history of depression, both of which increase her risk of becoming depressed. She is still being treated for her most recent depression. She has stressors in her relationship and in her job. Ms. B has a personal and family history of bipolar disorder but is not on maintenance mood stabilizers. Ms. C has a diagnosis of schizophrenia that, untreated, could flare up during pregnancy. All three are wise to come for prenatal counselling and advice regarding management in pregnancy.

Preconception planning

Prevention of mental health problems during pregnancy should begin in preconception. Any woman should have access to necessary supports during pregnancy. Ideally, the obstetrician or midwife is aware of risk factors for a woman requiring more support during this time. If necessary, she may require referral to a counsellor or a psychiatrist who has expertise in perinatal mental health.

Support is an important component of women staying well during pregnancy. If there are marital or family conflicts, ideally the patient can be helped to deal with these or be directed to counselling. Failing that, other resources should be recommended. Often, public health programs have groups or programs designed to provide available resources for women who feel alone or who are emotionally struggling. Social workers may be able to help with financial advice or resources for those struggling with these types of stressors. There should be a circle of care that includes doctors treating any other physical illness the patient has so that everyone understands the need to provide optimal care and support.

For those women with a history of major depression, anxiety or substance abuse or disorders such as bipolar disorder, schizophrenia or other psychiatric illnesses, preconception planning is essential. Women who have been taking medication for any of these illnesses should be educated as to the risk/benefit of taking medication during pregnancy. Fortunately, most psychiatric medications are safe during pregnancy. On the other hand, just stopping medication creates a high chance of risking a relapse during the pregnancy with added complications for the woman and the baby. Women should not merely be told to take medication but should be educated as to the research indicating the safety of most psychiatric medications and the risks both to her and the baby of not taking medication.

Psychological support and counselling or cognitive behavior therapy may be important components of prenatal care to help the woman deal with personal psychological stressors.

In summary, there are many risk factors for developing mental health problems during pregnancy. These include: A personal or family history of depression, anxiety, or other major psychiatric illness; current stressors; physical problems during pregnancy; lack of support systems; and traumatic pregnancies or deliveries. Non-traditional pregnancies in transgendered men or non-binary individuals bring another layer of possible external stress. Assessing these risk factors prior to pregnancy allows interventions to decrease the risk with support, counselling and, when indicated, medication. The aim of all of these interventions is to decrease the risk of major mental health problems and increase the chance of an enjoyable pregnancy and postpartum.

Dr. Gail Erlick Robinson is a Professor of Psychiatry and Obstetrics/Gynaecology at the University of Toronto and Co-founder of the Women's Mental Health Program at the University of Toronto. She has a special interest in the psychological impact of various aspects of women's reproductive life. In 2017, she received the Order of Canada for her work concerning the mental and physical health of women and regulation of the health professions. Connect with Dr. Robinson on Twitter @DrGailRobinson

IF I HAD ONE WISH

Sandra Pomar

I SQUEEZE MY EYES SHUT, hoping and praying the pregnancy test I just took will be positive.

Slowly I see the letters forming.

P-R-E-G-N-A-N-T

Pregnant?

I'M PREGNANT!

I'm ecstatic, but I don't tell anyone yet, not even my husband. I want to make sure I am 100% pregnant.

I run out to get more pregnancy tests, four more—two digital and two old school, the kind where you have to guess if the extremely faint line means you're pregnant or not.

I take all four tests and sure enough, they all confirm that, yes, I am pregnant! Now I can tell my husband and make an appointment with my doctor to confirm it.

Again.

A few days later, I'm spotting. Google reassures me that it's just implantation bleeding. I need to know for sure. I get yet another pregnancy test. If my husband knew the amount of money I've been spending on pregnancy tests, he'd have a fit.

I'm still pregnant. Thank goodness.

Four days later, I am at my doctor's to get a blood and urine test. The blood test will take a couple days to get the results, but the urine test comes back right away. When I first get to his office, I tell him the tale of all the pregnancy tests I've taken and how overjoyed my husband and I are to be pregnant but now, on his way back into the office with the results of the urine test, I see a look of bafflement cross his face. The test has come back negative.

My heart sinks. I want to vanish behind the walls and never be seen again. I am so confused and upset because I spent over $100 on tests and

I was pregnant, wasn't I? I have always used these tests, and they were always correct. I have other children to prove it!

So what is different now? After pleading with my doctor to recheck the test, he does and says there is a very faint line but we should wait for the results of the blood test before confirming one way or another.

I take the faint line as a sign that yes, indeed, I am still pregnant. Thank goodness. At this point, I can't bear the thought of not being pregnant. But I leave the doctor's office with some doubt.

I can't wait for the results of the blood test. I need to know, so I buy more tests. My husband comes into the bedroom and asks why I have more tests lying across the bed. I tell him it's just to see how the pregnancy is progressing. He seems to be okay with this excuse.

Just like the first time I took the first test, I squeeze my eyes shut and hope and pray the test is positive. The letters begin to form.

N-O-T P-R-E-G-N-A-N-T

I run down the stairs crying to my husband. He simply says not to worry, that I was being silly taking all those tests.

I need answers. I google. I read that I've either having a miscarriage or I simply took the test too late at night.

Too late at night? Is that a thing? I cling to the last bit of hope I have that I might still be pregnant.

Unfortunately, a few days later, after spending an insane amount of money on even more pregnancy tests, I officially miscarry. So I can now confirm that I was indeed pregnant and now I'm not. I instantly feel an overwhelming sense of loss.

My heart is completely crushed. I cry all day. My other children wonder what's wrong. I tell them I am sick. I need help, mental health help, but with it being a weekend there's nowhere to go except the emergency department. I decide to tell my children the truth, because I simply can't cope mentally on my own. They each place a teddy bear on my pillow, saying they are for "baby."

If I could have one wish, it would be to invent a pregnancy test that could reassure women that we won't miscarry and that everything will be okay. Is that wishful thinking? The anxiety that we moms go through when a miscarriage happens is all-consuming. No one else can ever comprehend the immense tension we feel in the first few weeks and months of pregnancy.

No matter how many children you currently have, no matter how far along you are, it's still a loss, a being that could have been.

I just want my baby back.

Sandra Pomar is a mom of five and lives in Alberta, Canada. She has worked as an educator in Quebec, Alberta, and the U.K. Her mission and desire in life is to help children worldwide experience laughter and joy. You can find Sandra on Instagram @Busydisneymama, on Twitter @pomar_sandra and she writes on her blog at http://Busydisneymama.simplesite.com/

BORN STILL

Nadine Belzile

When she was in my womb, Judith was doing kickboxing, that much was obvious. She was full of energy, was moving frequently and was kicking hard. At 37 weeks pregnant, I started noticing that my kickboxing baby was moving less frequently and kicking less hard. Though slightly worried, I decided to wait a few days to speak with my doctor during my routine scheduled appointment. The doctor listened to a few heartbeats and told me it was normal to feel the baby move less towards the end of pregnancy. Reassured, I returned home.

Two days later, I could no longer feel my baby move. My husband and I made our way to the hospital, but it was already too late; Judith's heart had stopped beating. I delivered a baby girl, stillborn at 38 weeks of pregnancy. The autopsy report revealed that Judith was healthy and died from asphyxia, i.e., lack of oxygen caused by an inflammation of the umbilical cord. I now know that had I gone to the hospital a week sooner, my little Judith would probably be alive today.

The social worker who visited me at the hospital gave me the name of a perinatal loss support group in my city, which met on a monthly basis. Each month welcomed new parents having gone through traumatic miscarriages or stillbirths. I felt my husband and I were not alone in our struggles. In parallel, I reconnected with a psychologist I had consulted in the past, though it took me a few months before I had the courage to do so. I was lucky to have the support of my husband and family through the whole ordeal. But even with all this positive support, I was not able to escape the devastating mental health problems that followed.

I spent the first five months following Judith's death in a haze, crying all day, every day. I was unable to take care of my three-year-old son. My husband had to do everything in the house; I was completely nonfunctional. Because Judith was born still, I no longer had access to 34 weeks of parental leave, which meant I had to go back to work after 18 weeks of maternity leave. I lasted four days. I experienced uncontrollable bursts of crying on each of those days. I remember, on the fourth day, sitting in a meeting room with my colleagues and having flashbacks of the hospital room in which I gave birth. That's when I realized I was struggling with post-traumatic stress disorder (PTSD).

I tried contacting my family doctor, but she was on vacation at the time, so I decided my best course of action was to go to the emergency room to get psychiatric help. I remember sitting in the waiting room and hearing babies cry. My head was filled with their cries and I started to cry myself, bent over the chair, holding my sides. My husband and I had to leave the waiting room and go wait a little further down the corridor.

I spent the night at the hospital under observation and, the next day, was transferred to the psychiatric ward where I spent a week and a half. I was diagnosed with severe major depression and PTSD. When I was discharged, I had a psychiatrist assigned to me.

I was lucky I had access to long-term disability leave at my workplace. It took me a total of nine months before I was ready to gradually go back to work. It took me another year before I was back at work full time. And that's when I became pregnant with my third child.

The pregnancy was very stressful as I was fearful of losing my baby at any time. I went back on disability leave after six months. I went through another traumatic birth, as I had to be rushed into surgery for an emergency C-section. Thankfully, my son was born alive and healthy. But depression and PTSD symptoms came back in full force during the months that followed. My family doctor diagnosed me with severe post-partum depression. I asked her to take over my treatment as I no longer wanted to be treated by the psychiatrist that had been assigned to me in the hospital. The man kept saying my daughter was probably better off dead because she was sick and that it was not helpful to keep pictures of her. I couldn't deal with his comments any more.

When I returned to work full-time, I thought I was fine, but a few months later, I had to start cutting back on my work hours as I was struggling with stress, anxiety, and fatigue. I started having panic attacks on a daily basis. My family doctor put me on medical leave, and I have never returned to work since. I realized then that I needed to deal with my PTSD symptoms, but my family doctor and my psychologist seemed to shy away from the issue. So I decided to venture out on my own and found a therapist specialized in Eye Movement Desensitization and Reprocessing (EMDR), a promising treatment for PTSD. I spent a year in therapy, and I rarely have panic attacks anymore. Thanks to my family doctor, I also got access to a new psychiatrist who adjusted my medication and had me follow two group therapies for depression and anxiety. Nonetheless, I continue to this day to struggle on and off with anxiety, depression and PTSD, and with taking care of myself and my family.

No parent should live through the death of their baby if that death can be prevented. All Canadian women should be empowered with the knowledge and confidence to prevent stillbirth.

Nadine Belzile holds an M.A. in anthropology and worked for 15 years as a research and public policy analyst for the Government of Canada. She is the mother of two boys and a stillborn daughter. Nadine developed Canada's first-ever website, www.BabyKicks.ca, (in French at www.BebeBouge.ca) dedicated to fetal movement counting during the third trimester as a means of preventing stillbirth. Nadine initiated a petition asking the Government of Canada to follow the lead of other countries and take action to end preventable stillbirths in Canada. Connect with Nadine on Twitter @BBougeBabyKicks

UNTIL WE SEE THE LIGHT

Alexandra Lihou

* *For this article I am using she, her, hers, and mom pronouns. However, it is important to recognize and honour my non-binary, gender nonconforming, and genderqueer clients.*

I was a new grad when I began working in the reproductive mental health program eight years ago. The program consisted of a registered clinical counsellor two-and-a-half days a week, a psychiatrist, who worked three days a week, and me. At the beginning, we did not accept grief clients. Writing that now, and now knowing what I do, it seems absurd. However, we just didn't have the capacity. We consulted and provided treatment for mothers that were struggling with new or pre-existing mental health concerns in pregnancy or in the postpartum period. But then a patient's baby was born still.

I remember so vividly sitting at my desk, preparing for our upcoming session—the first follow-up after her baby was born. We had worked together for months, we prepared a birthing plan that navigated not only her physical but psychological and emotional needs. I pulled up her electronic file excitedly and saw the little yellow baby carriage icon that indicates that the patient's baby was born. I began reading her labour and delivery notes as I wanted to be prepared to process her birth with her. As I read, my heart sank. Shock set in that her baby had died.

I walked out to our waiting room to collect her and when my eyes landed on her, I knew that everything had changed. A massive shift in her presence. Her light had dimmed. Slowly, she told me through her shock and disbelief what had happened. We sat and cried together. I apologized for crying, because historically, I was told never to cry with a patient, that crying hijacked my patient's experience and made it about me. However, at that moment she welcomed my tears. She knew that I was invested, connected, and she and her little one mattered. She also taught me that I was woefully underprepared to support her. As a therapist, I was capable of providing grief therapy, but this was different. This was traumatic grief, and I knew that I had to refer her to a more capable therapist. I was heartbroken. I felt like I had failed her.

I began to question what was happening to the grieving parents. Who was supporting them? Where were they referred? Because it certainly wasn't to me. I had been naive about how often babies were not compatible with life outside the womb, born too early, born still, or passed soon after birth. That, when a pregnancy is interrupted, regardless of the reason, there is often deep grief that follows. The more I researched, the more disheartened I became. I was bewildered that there were very few specialized reproductive grief clinicians in our area. And so many parents were struggling. I connected with the social work team in maternity and the NICU. I began reading books on grief. I focused all of my continuing education on grief and attended perinatal grief seminars. I was warned by a colleague that this was a path to burnout. She asked if I really want to put myself through this. "Umm, Yes," was my gut response. I knew I had to be properly prepared and educated, and so I became a compassionate bereavement care certified provider.

Dr. Joanne Cacciatore, bereaved mother, founder of the MISS Foundation for families experiencing the death of a child, Doctor of Psychology and professor, shares that 75% of grief therapy is grief education. The other 25% is holding a safe and compassionate space for the grieving process to unfold.

Loss of an infant or loss during pregnancy is often traumatic, sudden, and unexpected. In my work, I support individuals and families who grieve due to infertility, miscarriage, stillbirth, pregnancy interruption, and infant loss. I am a companion on their grief journey. I sit with them in the darkness of their despair, disbelief, and anguish, until we eventually start to see the light.

In our work together, we give voice to and honor the parent's story with every intention to provide a safe, non-judgmental openness for the mother to process and make sense of her loss. And yes, regardless of how long the parent held their baby internally or in their arms, they are all parents. The parent shares the details of their reproductive experience. I want to honor her challenges with fertility, the details and experiences of her pregnancy, the birth of her little one, however the birth unfolds, and of her loss. We honor her loss. We use her baby's name. We look at photos and mementos of a life that wasn't able to be lived.

Her story is often riddled with impossible decisions that a new parent should never have to make. I sit with the parent in her questioning her decisions and of what happened. Often she takes on responsibility for the loss and feels guilt, shame, blame, anger, regret, and deep guttural sadness. She feels unfairness and ponders the unanswerable questions: *Why my baby? Why my body?* I do not rescue her from her lived experience, I take her deeper into it. To rescue is to minimize. Thought-challenging is futile. One cannot think their way out of grief. We need to feel all the feelings—pushing them down will only lead to them growing darker and more intense and will surely surface later.

We process to allow the brain to understand what has happened to her body. There is a brain/body disconnect that occurs with the traumatic death. We process to incorporate her loss into her life story, to honor the existence of her little one. There are often no answers as to why the loss has occurred, why the embryo or fetus was not compatible with life outside of her body. Rarely is the autopsy report definitive. We work to live in the uncomfortable and the unknown.

Often the family's loss has confirmed to them their desire to have a baby. Families that have suffered a loss are not deterred; they are often emboldened. Approximately 85% of women who have suffered a loss will be pregnant again within 18 months. But it is in my experience that most families continue trying to conceive again in approximately three to four months or as soon as they are medically cleared to do so. The desire to conceive is often met with intense worry and fear of history repeating, regardless of the optimism their primary-care team has conveyed. Our therapeutic work often transitions to anxiety management, allowing space for the potential new one in their narrative while honoring and remembering their loss. Although every journey is unique, it is in my experience that every single client that wants to grow their family does so, whether they birth from their own body, from that of a surrogate or through adoption.

Through my time supporting grieving individuals and families, I have observed a consistent pattern. Out of the brokenness grows a sense of self and a striving for purpose, not a reason for their loss but a call to duty so no one else has to feel or experience the pain that they have. The goal is often to support other parents who grieve and to reduce the chance of a similar loss from occurring in the future.

As a companion on their grief journey, I have learned so very much from my clients. I am often in awe of their strength and resilience. I have come to recognize that the act of advocating is the individual taking back control following a time where they felt deep helplessness. This can happen in many different ways, from supporting friends or acquaintances who are newly bereaved, joining a local bereavement group, publishing the story of their loss, joining a butterfly run or fundraising initiatives to support bereaved families, and petitioning local members of parliament for increased support for bereaved families in their community.

I am often invited by my clients to advocate with them. We have taken part in TV interviews where clients have shared their stories in the effort to reduce the stigma of mental health during the grieving process. We have petitioned the Government of Canada through Motion 110, a study of the impact on parents who have suffered the loss of an infant or child. And I have spoken as a witness to the Standing Committee on Human Resources, Skills and Social Development in the House of Commons, advocating for a parental bereavement benefit to provide financial support at a time where the costs are numerous and the pressure to return to work is unethical.

Being a reproductive grief therapist is an honour, and I do my work with loving gratitude for my clients. Dr. Joanne Cacciatore speaks of a "civic love" that forms between herself and her clients. Civic love is the love for one's community and a commitment to the common good. It is impossible to do this work and not form a civic love for those bereaved in our community.

Alexandra Lihou is a Compassionate Bereavement Certified Provider and a Perinatal Mental Health Certified Counsellor. Connect with Alexandra on Instagram @holding_space_for_women

CAN'T STOP CRYING

Jena Andaya

NO ONE LIKES TO SPEAK about how dark a mind can get, about how you can wake up without the desire to carry on.

I am told early on by our very kind family doctor that many health practitioners will try to call my pregnancy at age 39, a geriatric pregnancy, and that I should prepare myself to hear these words. Dr. K explains that it comes from a need to be upfront with a patient so they are aware of the complications and are able to manage outcomes better. It still stings when I first hear my obstetrician say it. And then she adds another lacklustre title to the mix, *advanced maternal age pregnancy.*

I cry. I can't stop crying. *What is happening to me?*

Thankfully, I have a husband who never fails to reassure me that I am built to do this and a parent who reminds me often how blessed I am. I have siblings who never waver in their love for me and the little life I carry in my belly, friends who drop everything to come to my aid, and health care practitioners who always show me genuine empathy and direction.

Still, my mind gets dark.

Some days, it takes all I have just to get through one task. I don't understand what's happening to me. In a room full of people I know and love, I feel alone. Fear often overcomes me and takes over. I notice that I am making careless mistakes at work. It's taking so much effort to focus. I can't stay present and engaged in my relationship with my husband, and as supportive as he is, it begins to take a toll on our marriage.

At one of my obstetrician appointments, I break down. In between sobs, I apologize, saying I know he probably had a busy day but I don't know who else to turn to. I feel so defeated. The doctor gives me a referral to see a psychiatrist.

At my initial psychiatric appointment, I am asked to fill out the Edinburgh Postnatal Depression Scale. My score is high. At 36 weeks pregnant, I am diagnosed with perinatal anxiety and depression. The psychiatrist explains what our plan will be going forward—medication, psychotherapy, self-care, and exercise. She gives me a few leads on private non-profits in the area where I might turn to for more counselling and support.

I leave her office worrying about how I am going to explain a diagnosis of prenatal depression and anxiety to my husband. How am I going to explain it to my siblings? In an immigrant culture where mental illness is never spoken of, never acknowledged, I know I have to tread lightly.

My husband is very confused but tries his best to understand. We have been trying to get pregnant for a little more than a year, and this is supposed to be a happy time for us. Ultimately, he tells me, "Whatever comes, we will get through it, together."

My family on the other hand, is less than supportive. I am pained at hearing them tell me that I have finally gone crazy, that I am attention seeking, and a disappointment. In most South Asian cultures, a mental illness is viewed as a weakness and an embarrassment. Even worse, it is something you do not speak of or burden family with.

To this day, we never speak of my diagnosis.

Jena lives in Regina, Saskatchewan with her husband and son, where she forgets to water all their house plants. Please don't tell her husband.

MY HYPEREMESIS HYPER-NEMESIS

Emily Pollak

My husband and I want to have two children and we're so excited when we learn about our rainbow pregnancy.

But the excitement is short-lived.

By six weeks, morning sickness starts with a vengeance and I am diagnosed with hyperemesis gravidarum which causes severe nausea and vomiting during pregnancy.

I go from an being an active mom to completely incapacitated and I have to take a medical leave from work.

The vomiting and nausea are so intense, I move my beanbag chair into the bathroom. My bathroom becomes my primary living space. I'm not able to eat or drink or have any sensory input.

I reach out to my family doctor. Her advice is to eat crackers. I am dropping weight quickly and I'm starving. I feel like I have the worst stomach bug that never seems to end. The vomiting is forceful, and I have vomited all the stomach bile I have. My esophagus burns. I know I need help and I need it quickly. My family doctor is useless and unfortunately, the way the health care system is set up, obstetricians do not start care until 12 weeks in pregnancy.

It's Christmas Eve and I need medical care. I spend the day in the emergency room getting fluids and then I'm discharged home but the vomiting continues. I am lightheaded, dizzy, weak, my lips are parched, and my stomach hurts from all the vomiting. Needless to say, I feel awful.

Christmas is supposed to be a wonderful time of year and I want to celebrate the magic with my two-year-old son, but I am bedridden. With the support of my mom and with many breaks to catch my breath, I muster up the strength in my body to move. I am able to make it down the stairs. I passively watch my son open gifts and have a moment of joy but that quickly leaves as the physical symptoms remain at the forefront of my battle.

I return to the emergency room on Boxing Day, pleading for help. The doctor gives me another IV treatment and again discharges me with no follow-up plans in place.

I feel so alone. I am reaching out for support, but no one is able to give me what I need, which is relief. I can't think about living day to day, it's minute to minute. I am trying to survive. I share with others about my pregnancy in the hopes of getting support. However, I am met with congratulations and excitement, but that is far from how I am feeling. I want this baby so badly after having had a miscarriage, but there are moments I beg for it to stop. I am robbed of joy.

The symptoms are so severe, no one can eat or bring take-out food into the home or I will vomit. If my husband has coffee and comes near me, I will vomit. If I watch TV, I will vomit. All I can do is lie in my bed, in the dark silence. If I need to use the washroom, my mom comes with me, carrying my IV bags. If I need to bathe, my mom helps undress and bathe me. I have lost all my dignity and privacy and have become dependent on the care of others. This is not what I imagined pregnancy to be like.

Worst of all, no one is taking charge of my medical care. I decide to visit an early pregnancy clinic where I can be monitored. They set up home health care so I can receive 24/7 IV therapy. At the clinic, the doctors perform an ultrasound and reassure me that my baby is doing great. What they neglect to see is that I am not doing great. The hyperemesis gravidarum is taking a toll on not just my body but also my mind.

My son misses me, and I miss him. I am not able to be the mom I want to be for him. I am forced to abruptly wean him. He has a little toy house with a doorbell and pretends to be a nurse ringing the bell to care for mommy. It breaks my heart.

I begin to have heart palpitations from malnutrition, and my anxiety increases. I feel scared and worry that I'm going to die in my sleep. I have gone over a month without a bowel movement. The visiting nurse tries to stay upbeat, but I become a human pin cushion. Eventually, all my veins blow out, and I am no longer able to get my IV medication.

I am at a loss and try to research my next steps. I read that I may need a PICC line, which is a catheter that is inserted in a peripheral vein in the arm that is guided to a larger vein that eventually leads to the heart.

I have exhausted my options with the temporary IVs and might need this next step. I follow-up with the early pregnancy clinic and after multiple phone calls, they write a script for a PICC line. Unfortunately, they do not set up the procedure for me, and I have to go back to the emergency room to get it inserted. In the operating room, a team of doctors and nurses surround me and insert the PICC line into my vein. It feels surreal. This is my pregnancy.

Although I now have the PICC line, the drug being inserted into my body is not controlling the hyperemesis gravidarum. I feel mentally drained, and I need help. Unfortunately, my family doctor is absent and the early pregnancy clinic is only focused on the baby. I need someone to help me. I need a doctor to recognize the severity of the situation and not pass me off to the next doctor or clinic or emergency room.

I find a nurse practitioner, Jadie, who is able to see me quickly. Jadie is my miracle. She is what I needed from the beginning. Jadie sees me; she sees that I am suffering. She recognizes that this is traumatic for me. I have gone from a healthy 155-pound woman to 120 pounds in six weeks. She quickly springs into action and has me admitted to the hospital.

Being admitted to the hospital is the last thing that I want, but it is what I need. It is my first time away from my son, and my heart shatters. He cries without me, and my mom and husband try to comfort and soothe him.

The hospital stay is not easy, but it is worth it. There are some nurses that tell me because I am less than 20 weeks pregnant, that I shouldn't be in their unit because they don't want to provide complex care. I don't know why they are telling me this, and it makes me feel alone and guilty. There are a few wonderful nurses who come and keep me company.

The chief obstetrician takes over my care. He advocates within the labour and delivery unit for me to be treated with professionalism and respect as my illness is pregnancy-related. He is finally able to get my condition under control with a cocktail of medications. I am able to have the PICC line painfully removed from my arm, as the nurses gently pull it out. I am finally able to eat, and I have some chicken soup and begin to take medication orally.

Pulling into my driveway and seeing my son greet me is such an emotional moment. I am relieved to be home after my two-week hospital stay, and I'm feeling more like myself. I have a long road to recovery as I need to build my body strength back after months of bed rest. I build my circle of support, I see a pelvic floor physiotherapist, a chiropractor, a naturopath, and a massage therapist. Each one of them provides me with such compassionate care. I am forever grateful to my circle of care team including Jadie and the chief obstetrician.

I decide to hire a doula to support me through my birth as my pregnancy was so traumatic. During my labour, my baby is in distress and his heart rate is dropping. The next thing I know, staff are running into my room, and a nurse is shouting at me to push. I feel a moment of fear, but then lock eyes with my doula. She is my safe person, and she brings me comfort.

I push for twenty minutes, and my son is born. He is swollen and puffy but okay. I had gone through so much to bring him into this world, and at last here he is, safe in my arms. The hyperemesis gravidarum is gone and my baby is here. Now, I can focus on being a mom and caring for my infant. Unfortunately, though the hyperemesis gravidarum is physically gone, what I went through has left mental and emotional scars that I carry with me post-pregnancy.

My postpartum journey is filled with severe anxiety. I am terrified that something awful will happen to a member of my family. My anxiety is related to the health and safety of my children. I am hyper-vigilant with any symptoms that resemble an illness. I am scared travelling in the car. I have intrusive thoughts about being hit and dying in a car accident. I am scared that something will happen to my baby and I will not be able to help him. I feel alone in these feelings as others do not seem to understand me. I am constantly on edge and start to wonder if all this is a result of my traumatic pregnancy.

I do more research and learn that over half of hyperemesis gravidarum survivors experience trauma-related symptoms, such as avoidance, numbing, hypervigilance, the re-experiencing sensations, and being easily triggered by distressing reminders of what happened. I am suffering from post-traumatic stress disorder.

I suffer in silence. I'm afraid of how others will perceive me if I tell them about the intrusive thoughts I'm having. I am afraid someone will think that I am a bad mom. Having worked as a former child protection worker, I am also traumatized by what I've experienced there, and I'm afraid that if I tell a friend about how I'm feeling, they will call child services.

I decide to see a psychiatrist who, thankfully, is so kind and accepting of me. She adjusts the antianxiety medication I had been taking throughout pregnancy and postpartum and provides me with bi-weekly psychotherapy. She reassures me that I am a good mom, and that I am not a child protection concern. It takes me some time to build trust and believe that is the truth.

Healing has not been linear. It has been a bit of a rollercoaster. There are still parts I am working through five years later, like trusting healthcare providers. There are some foods I will never eat, as they are still a strong reminder of that difficult time.

It is from this lived experience, however, that I've decided to help change the world of perinatal mental health. I decided to leave my job in child protection and dedicate my career to maternal mental health. I'm so glad I made this decision. It is from the combination of my professional training and lived experience that I am proud to have become a well-known psychotherapist in my area. I have built a team of health care providers in an effort to streamline services, so no one is ever alone.

Emily Pollak is a mom of two and lives in the Niagara region of Ontario. She is a registered social worker and the owner of Maternal Health Niagara, which provides perinatal wellness services. Emily's vision is building a circle of support for individuals and families during the reproductive period and beyond. Emily's clinical focus is infertility, pregnancy loss, pregnancy, birth trauma, postpartum anxiety, and postpartum depression. She coaches women through "mom guilt" and managing the mental load of motherhood. You can find Emily on Facebook and Instagram @MaternalNiagara

BIRTH TRAUMA

Bonnie Burns

IT'S SIX AM. MY CONTRACTIONS start. I manage them throughout the day until we decide it's time to go to the hospital. The pain has stretched all around my back and up my spine. I don't want an epidural, but at three centimetres dilation, the contractions are intense and close.

"Give me the drugs!" I say to the nurse, and in less than ten minutes, I am feeling great.

And then I'm not feeling so great.

I start to feel nauseous, and the colour drains from my face. My husband sees that my blood pressure drops to half what it was. The next thing I know, I'm throwing up and surrounded by nurses and the doctor.

I'm unplugged from the machines and am being wheeled into the operating room. I'm dizzy, so dizzy. I can hear the doctor firing off orders to the nurses. Turns out I am in the operating room in case I need an emergency C-section.

I wait, helpless on the gurney, with no visual of my husband. Nurses are running around the room, getting things in order. The doctor is talking to me, but all I want to know is whether my baby is okay. I feel panic running through me, sweat building up, and another wave of nausea. I know I need to calm down. I need to breathe.

I search the room and find the heart rate monitor. I lock eyes on it. I feel my husband beside me and his hands wrap around mine. I can see that my heart rate and that of our baby's are both steadying, and I find comfort in watching the numbers level. Finally, we stabilize and get the okay to go back to the birthing room. A sigh of relief washes over me, and all I feel are tears welling up in my eyes. I swallow the knot in my throat and think, not yet, I still need to birth our baby, and I need to be strong. Don't cry.

In the birthing room, the nurses hook me back up to the machines, and we play the waiting game. I am now five centimetres dilated and the doctor decides that we are going to try Oxytocin at half the dosage to stimulate contractions. I am exhausted, both mentally and physically. I have been in active labour for 12 hours now and I haven't eaten and I feel like I don't have any energy left.

The nurse can see my exhaustion and tells my husband that I need to get some rest. As I am in and out of sleep, the doctor and nurses come in and out of the room. I turn my head to look at the heart monitor and see that my baby's heart rate is dropping again. This time, it's from the Oxytocin.

The nurses flip me from my right to my left, and back again, trying to get the baby's heart rate up. Finally, once again, she stabilizes. At this point, my water has yet to break. I am still stuck at five centimetres. The doctor decides to break my water, and says it's time for the full dose of Oxytocin now. If I don't fully dilate, they'll be wheeling me back to the operating room for a C-section.

I am so sad, not that I might have to get a C-section, but because I feel like my body is failing me and my baby. Why does her heart rate keep dropping? I feel a wave of nausea rising back up in my throat. My baby's heart rate starts to lower even further. There's more flipping me from right to left. My baby's heart rate lowers even further and then, it stops.

The nurse rushes to get the doctor. Moments later, the doctor enters the room with four nurses following quickly behind her. A flood of tears well up in my eyes again, and this time I can't stop them.

"Enoughs enough!" the doctor says, "It's time to get that baby out of there!"

I'm handed forms to sign as the nurses begin unplugging me from the machines again and wheeling me out the door all in a matter of seconds. The flashback of being wheeled down the same corridor just a few hours ago creates a pit in my stomach, as I re-live the anxiety again.

We get to the operating room, and my husband has to stay back and wait until everything is set up before he can go in. I've never felt so alone and scared. As I lay there, I watch the team prep, and all I can think about is keeping our baby safe. Another wave of nausea comes and the anesthesiologist grabs a bin and comforts me as I throw up into it. I keep reciting in my head, *she's going to be okay, just breathe.*

Finally the curtain goes up, and my husband is able to join me. I've held the tears back all day, but I can't anymore. Everything comes pouring out. My husband grabs my hand, leans in close to my face, and whispers, "Everything's going to be okay. I love you. She's going to be here soon."

The tears keep streaming down my face, but I believe him. My husband, my rock, gives me the extra strength I need to keep pushing through, and the next thing we know, the doctor shouts, "Get your camera ready!"

And then I hear the sweetest sound, a baby crying, our baby girl crying. She is finally here. She is okay. The tears of fear and sadness transform to a flood of relief and joy.

My husband cuts the umbilical cord, and the nurse brings our baby over to me. She puts her on the bed right by my face, and her little face stares back at me. She is here. She is safe. She is healthy. She is perfect. As they finish sewing me up, the doctor comes up to my bed and says, "Great job, mama. You did it! She's here, and she's beautiful."

I thought I prepared for everything for the birth, but nothing could've prepared me for what had just happened. The healing both physically and mentally from the birth events takes a while. I keep thinking my body failed me and that I should've been strong enough to take the pain and bypass the epidural. The *what ifs* haunt me. What if it hadn't turned out the way it did? It's been almost two years, and I still think about it. I think I always will.

Bonnie Burns is a mom of one and lives in Toronto. She strongly believes that the mental wellness of a mother matters, and now is the time to make that known. You can find Bonnie on Instagram @Mombrain_n_spitstains

Part 2:

Postpartum Depression & Anxiety

We Broke Mummy

We thought we'd broken Mummy,
She was lying on the floor.
Tears were streaming down her face.
Big tears just like before.

We thought we'd broken Mummy,
We'd heard her shout and scream.
Maybe she was angry or
She'd had a nasty dream.

We thought we'd broken Mummy,
She stayed in bed all day
Just staring at her bedroom walls.
She didn't come and play.

We thought we'd broken Mummy,
She didn't look the same.
She didn't sing or play along,
until a lady came.

We thought we'd broken Mummy,
Until she made us chips for tea.
A picnic on the carpet
Just for our family.

We hadn't broken Mummy,
'She could just do with some rest.
Her brain is full of spinning plates
And she feels a bit depressed.'

We hadn't broken Mummy,
But she still needs some time to heal.
Those spinning plates of mental health
Aren't visible but they're real.

Leander Moore
@postpartumpoet

DAY NINE

Amanda Munday

WHAT WILL HAPPEN TO ME this time, now that I've revealed my crumbling mind to others? What happens when other people find out I'm not managing parenthood well? Without the option to sleep or take a break from my responsibilities, the threat of death seems more real today. It's probably because I'm about to die.

The sense of urgency to get to the hospital and have someone confirm my broken mental state is palpable. *I feel the rush to be seen and diagnosed rising behind my ears. My back is stiff, and my stomach is in a nervous knot. If I go to the hospital, I'll have a few hours where I can't hurt the baby. Where I can't lose control. Maybe there will be air conditioning in the ER, too, and I can get some relief from this bloody humidity. I will be safe there.*

Once we're packed up, with my sister in the front seat and me in the back with the baby, I realize that this is the first time I've been in the car since we brought her home from the hospital. It's 9:30 p.m. on this hot summer weeknight and the sun is just starting to set. *This tiny baby has to come along to see her mother be assessed for madness.* I realize I've missed the summer solstice. Irony lingers between the longest day of the year and the longest week of my existence.

We drive along the quiet side streets and the city exhales. Being out of the house feels almost whimsical, like resolution. I lean my head against the window and I sway side to side with each turn onto a new street. The baby sleeps in her bucket seat beside me. I grab her tiny hand.

"Your Mama is going to get better, my love. This is how I get better."

Doubts resurface. *I shouldn't have asked my family to do this for me. They're heading to an emergency room on a Thursday night because I begged them to. I feel a bit better. Should I tell them I feel a bit better? Maybe all I needed was a car ride.* The relief is sweet, but I still sense it's unstable, like the meringue on top of gelatinous lemon pie. I remember that we didn't bring anything but a diaper bag.

I walk into the emergency room and carry the baby to the triage desk. A nurse waves me over immediately, and I have to quickly explain that we're not here because of the baby.

"The baby's fine. The baby is fine but I am not fine." I have tears in my eyes and a lump in my throat. She tells me to sit down beside her desk and begins asking me the basic registration details.

"What brings you to the ER tonight?"

I look up at my sister and husband and ask them to walk away from me. Alice is puzzled, and Gordon outright refuses to move. I want to protect them from the forthcoming details. But when I realize they aren't leaving, I tell the nurse what's happening through a stream of sobs and whines.

"Please help me. I can't sleep. I'm so scared. I don't know what's going on but I'm begging you to find someone who can help me understand what's happening to me."

I give her the quiet details of the phone cable and of the plastic bag. She asks me when I had a baby.

"Last Tuesday."

She counts on her fingers. "One...two...she's nine days old? Is that right? Did you hurt the baby?"

No? "No. The baby is fine. It's me who is not fine." I look over to Gordon, who is listening to this conversation with alert eyes, but ones I can see are exhausted. Did he expect his wife to be so crazy so soon after giving birth? My heart shatters looking at how tired he is, while I'm asking him to stand here and listen to my dark thoughts. I look back at the nurse and she's crying. She bites her lip and turns to face the computer monitor.

"Okay, have a seat. Someone will see you soon. You did the right thing." I'm telling myself that I did the right thing, but the truth is all I feel is regret. Regret that we're in the hospital on a Thursday night, regret that I'm not experiencing motherhood the way I thought I would, regret that I've stolen Gordon's experience as a new father. I'm devastated that nothing is going the way I thought it would. Do I deserve what is happening to me? *Why didn't I think this was a legitimate risk when I was pregnant? Why didn't I better prepare for this?*

Together we return to the waiting room. My husband, my sister, my baby, and me. Alice doesn't have a sweater. I didn't put on a bra before I left the house, and I realize my hair, pulled into a haphazard ponytail, makes me look even more erratic. We sit down in front of a man who's bleeding from his eyebrow. He smells of liquor and is shifting aggressively in his seat. Alice looks at me nervously, and Gordon says he's going to take the baby outside. I watch him wrap her in our new Moby carrier, freshly unpacked from my late-night Amazon order, and head outside. He walks back and forth between ambulances and taxis and I'm suddenly, but continuously, devastated.

Alice moves to a seat closer to me and says, "The doctor will make you feel better. Don't worry, okay?" She seems less confident than her words sound.

More taxis arrive to drop off ill patients. Flus, cuts, broken arms, a pregnant woman. Gordon holds both of his hands around Fiona's tiny ears to shield her from the sirens as he paces out front. A while later he heads back inside, and Fiona is crying. *Of course, I have to feed her.* This is the first time I'll attempt to breastfeed in public, and I couldn't feel more vulnerable and exposed. I'm sitting in an emergency room waiting area about to pull out my breast. *This place is full of illness. What if she contracts some cold or flu while we sit here? I am a neglectful parent.*

I struggle to get Fiona to latch. We aren't in our regular position, and the breastfeeding cover I have over my chest makes it difficult to see what's going on. An older woman stares at me. *She's looking at the nipple shield, judging my failures.* The man with the bleeding eyebrow is called in to see a doctor. *Was he here before me or after me? I'm losing track of time.*

It's now after midnight, and we are all exhausted. *Maybe I shouldn't have come. I've overreacted and don't need to be here.* When they finally call my name, we pack up the mobile baby office and follow the nurse behind the triage area and into the back hallway. We are led to the very back of the emergency area and brought into a small private room with a bed, a separate private washroom, and a side table. Emergency rooms don't usually come equipped with an en-suite washroom, so it strikes me as a little odd that I'd get this one. Is it to separate the baby from others, in case she cries and disturbs the sick patients? Before I can figure out why we are given the isolation room, a doctor enters.

"What's going on tonight?" Her tone is worn, and her gaze directed at Fiona. I look to my sister and ask her to leave again. The doctor, without looking at me, agrees that's a good idea, and asks Gordon and the baby to go with Alice into the hallway.

"There's a waiting area across the hall. We'll only be a few minutes."

I launch into the story, again. I explain that I feel like I'm dying. I haven't eaten in days and I'm not hungry. That I've been given opportunities to sleep but it doesn't happen. That I want to feel normal and I can't. That I haven't hurt the baby but I keep thinking I might. Racing thoughts. Intrusive thoughts. Terrible and disrupted nightmares when I do manage to sleep for a few minutes.

"What is going on with me? Please tell me what's wrong. Why do I feel this way?" I'm overwhelmed with grief, desperation, exhaustion, and fear. I dissolve into sobs. The doctor puts her hand on my shoulder and I slide away from her grasp. The gesture is kind, but I don't want to be touched, and I absolutely do not want to be touched by a stranger. She asked me about my labour and delivery, and all about what's happened over the last week.

Then she asks, "Is your husband hurting you? Are you here because you're in danger? Is the baby safe?"

The answer is yes, I'm in danger. But not because of my husband.

"You did the right thing coming here." She's the second person to tell me I did the right thing, so naturally I question it. *Are they saying it because I didn't really do the right thing and I'm wasting everyone's time?*

"I need to go and see another doctor; wait here. okay? I'll send your family back in." Gordon and Alice come back in with Fiona, and we all sit silently while I gulp back tears, not wanting to outright bawl in fear it will upset the baby. Gordon and Alice let out separate long exhales that sound a bit like emphatic sighs. We don't have anything to say to one another, so we simply wait. The doctor returns less than five minutes later presenting two pages of paperwork.

"I don't think you're going to leave, because you came here on your own today. But this is a document saying I want you to stay in the hospital for seventy-two hours. You have the right to get a court injunction to allow you to leave the hospital, but I don't think you're going to do that. This document says you're going to stay here and be observed, which I know you want to do to get better. Do you understand what I'm telling you? I will leave you with your copy of this document. Please review it."

I nod. What else can I do? I think she's saying I have to stay here for seventy-two hours. I guess that means I'm not going home tonight.

Gordon looks stunned and says nothing. I reach for Fiona and try unsuccessfully to feed her. Alice looks tired. This is her first exposure to our new reality, to the sleep deprivation and days that don't end. When I thought about what my new motherhood experience would look like, it didn't include bringing my sister to a psychiatric evaluation. It didn't include asking for help at all. This is her introduction to the night-is-day cycle, and it's a brutal orientation. With an exhausted plea, I say to Gordon, "Please take these two home. It's not safe for the baby here. She's going to get sick. You need to leave."

He resists. "I'm not leaving you in this fucking hospital. You just need some medication so you can sleep and you need to come home with me. Besides, you're her only food source. She wouldn't take a bottle before. I can't imagine going home without you and just hoping the baby magically starts feeding with a bottle. No way. You've never pumped and now you're just going to start using a pump? And store the milk where?"

"Listen," I say, "maybe if I'm not home, she'll drink from a bottle. What choice do we have? I don't know what to do either. The paperwork says I have to stay. We are out of options." I do my best to take charge of a situation I didn't see coming. "Go. Please? This is a ridiculous place for the baby to be."

We are arguing back and forth when an on-call psychologist bursts into my small shell of a room. When he moves the curtain back from around the bed, I see that I'm in a room surrounded by glass. The private washroom is here because I can't leave. *They can lock me in here. This is not a regular emergency room.* The doctor asks Gordon and my sister to leave again, but this time I hold onto the baby. I have to pinch my arm to remind myself that this doctor is a living, breathing human. He looks a bit like a caricature of a doctor. He's wearing a wrinkled black suit, a white shirt, and a black tie. The tie sits crookedly and loosely around his neck, an indication that he was called in specifically to see me and just threw these clothes on in a rush out the door. He must have been asleep. *He drew the short-straw on-call shift.*

He repeats the same questions: "Are you going to hurt yourself? Have you hurt the baby? Is there anyone in this room besides you, me, and the baby? Are you hearing voices? Do you believe the world is going to end? When was the last time you slept? Do you have a history of mental illness? What is your medical history? What happened at the birth? What do you want to happen next?"

"I'm really scared," I tell him.

"Why?" The doctor looks up from his notes.

"Well, because I'm sitting in a hospital after midnight talking to you about scary things. This is a pretty scary, messed-up situation." He smirks. I'm not sure why. More questions. He makes a few remaining notes, flipping the lined paper on his clipboard up and over.

"I'm going to go and speak with your husband and see what we can do about getting you a bed upstairs, okay? You did the right thing coming here."

I hear the doctor and Gordon talking outside my door.

"Your wife is still in there. She is not well, but I can tell she's somewhere inside there. I recommend she be sent upstairs where the doctors can monitor her 24/7 for a few days. You should discuss medication with them."

"How long is she going to have to stay here?" Gordon says. He's demolished; I can hear that much from behind the curtain.

"I don't know exactly, but I know it's safer here for her than at home," says the doctor. "You want your wife to get better, don't you? If you want her to get well, you need to leave her here. This is the safest place for her to be right now."

It's official: I'm in danger. Now I wish I was home but I can't leave. I'm a prisoner.

"Go home," I plead when Gordon walks back into the room. "They said I did the right thing."

Amanda Munday is a queer mom of two from Toronto, Ontario. She is an author and this selection originally appeared in her book, *Day Nine*, (Dundurn Press Limited, 2019) and appears here with her permission and that of Dundurn Press Limited. Find Amanda on Instagram @mundaywrites

INCLUSIVITY

Dr. Lesley A. Tarasoff

SOME PEOPLE WHO EXPERIENCE PREGNANCY, birth and parenting, and who seek perinatal care, including perinatal mental health care, do not identify as a mom or mother. Some people who experience pregnancy and birth do not identify as cisgender women or use the pronouns she and her. Relatedly, gender is not always a binary for people.

In recognition of people's diverse gender identities and expressions, many health organizations and authorities, such as the Canadian Association of Midwives [1], the Society of Obstetricians and Gynaecologists of Canada [2], and the Canadian Psychiatric Association [3], are increasingly making commitments to use gender-neutral or gender-inclusive language.

Using gender-inclusive language is important for several reasons.

In their study of transmasculine people's experiences feeding their newborns [4], MacDonald and colleagues importantly note that:

Language, both written and spoken, has power. Words can heal or wound, uplift or disparage....Being described with words such as she, her, mom, mum, mother, breasts, or breastfeeding could be distressing for a parent who self-identifies differently....Health care providers and others may inadvertently cause harm and intensify feelings of gender dysphoria by misgendering transmasculine patients. Conversely, care providers can affirm a patient's gender identity by gendering them correctly, and thus alleviate distress related to gender dysphoria.

It has also been noted that gendered language can be restrictive for more than just people who identify as trans, non-binary, or genderqueer [5]. Inclusive language also benefits many cisgender women who don't like being called "lady," who don't like checking the Ms, Mr, or Mrs box, or who don't want to be identified by their gender because they have experienced gender-based discrimination [5].

Inclusive language demonstrates a first step toward allyship on the part of friends and loved ones of trans or non-binary people [5] and justice for gender diverse communities broadly. Inclusive language helps us all to be more aware and sensitive to the devastating effects of marginalization [6]. Indeed, there is a growing body of research on the harmful impact of sexual and gender identity-based discrimination and stigma on the health of sexual and gender minority (or LGBTQ) people [7-10].

Sexual and gender minority people, and in particular bisexual women and trans people, experience high rates of mental illness [11-18]. There is growing evidence that sexual and gender minority people experience reproductive and perinatal health disparities, including perinatal mental health disparities [19-23]. Health-care practitioners may treat LGBTQ people who are pregnant differently than heterosexual and cisgender women based on pre-existing gender norms and assumptions about who should be able to experience pregnancy and birth (i.e., heterosexual, cisgender women) [24]. Trans and non-binary people are often misdiagnosed or dismissed by health care practitioners when expressing health concerns [24-25], and some LGBTQ people even delay or avoid accessing care due to anticipated discrimination or previous experiences of discrimination [25-29], which in turn may have an adverse impact their mental health [30].

Inclusive language helps us all to be more aware and sensitive to the needs of each family [6]. In efforts to support the mental health of pregnant people and parents in the perinatal period, we must recognize the diversity of family configurations (i.e., people form families and bring children into the world in a variety of ways, including using assisted reproduction or fertility services). As such, we must consider how different processes or experiences of family creation may affect mental health. Relatedly, we must be attentive to the mental health challenges and needs of the partners, non-birth parents, co-parents, and other biological and chosen family members and support persons. There is evidence, for example, that there are limited mental health services and supports for lesbian, bisexual, and queer non-birth parents [31]; as well, there is evidence that fathers, particularly first time fathers, experience depression during the perinatal period [32-33].

Using inclusive language is a small action to show respect and acknowledge diversity. Inclusive language creates more space for more people and that's better for everyone [38].

Dr. Lesley A. Tarasoff, PhD, is a Canadian Institutes of Health Research-funded Postdoctoral Research Fellow in the Department of Health and Society at the University of Toronto Scarborough and in the Azrieli Adult Neurodevelopmental Centre at the Centre for Addiction and Mental Health. She holds a PhD in Public Health Sciences, with a specialization in women's health, from the University of Toronto. For over a decade, she has been studying the reproductive, perinatal, and mental health of populations that are often stigmatized and marginalized, namely women with disabilities and sexual minority women. Find Dr. Tarasoff on Twitter @latarasoff

RELUCTANT LOVE

Parrish Wilson

I AM IN LOVE. BUT reluctantly.

There are moments when I look into this little baby's eyes and am awestruck that this person is *my* person. His eyes are my eyes. He came from my body, nourished by my milk, soothed by the feel of my skin against his as if we've always been one. Yet love and fear smash up against each other, and I feed the fear the most.

Because here, with my little person, I am desperately lonely.

Two weeks after his birth, my mother flies home and my partner goes back to work. The days are long. I'm not well enough, physically or emotionally, to get us out of the house.

Besides, you're not supposed to. New mommies and babies are supposed to stay home, rest, and be cared for so that they may focus just on each other, sleep and wake in unison, connected as they have always been. This has been the tradition in countless cultures around the world for all of history but not here, not in this life. In the Western world, we expect Mom to bounce back and be ready for outings and visitors, to go along with everyday life within a week or two.

Looking back, I believe a period of rest and nurturing would have led to a much different experience of early motherhood for me. It would have proven to me the importance of self-care, in asking for help and receiving it with grace. It would have given me the time to transition into motherhood with more love and compassion. It would have shown me the true importance of this role I was taking on. Permitting myself those quiet moments in bed with my baby, guilt-free, would have honoured the value of the work that I was going to do in caring for him as he grew. I would have felt less like just another woman who was coming up short—not pretty enough, not happy enough, not domesticated enough. I could have learned right away the magnitude of magic and power that is the essence of motherhood and nurturing life.

But instead, I busy myself because that's what modern women are taught to do when life gets tough. I cook and clean. I prepare to host Christmas a mere six weeks after giving birth. And in all the hustle and bustle, with my to-do list directing me, I get annoyed when a diaper needs changing or a nursing session takes an hour, followed by a two-hour nap in my arms, followed by another nursing session, leaving me stuck on the couch for an entire afternoon, unproductive, of sorts.

So I read and sleep, and stare out the window. And maybe it's a little bit like the rest every new mother and baby deserve, but it's riddled with guilt for not doing enough and with loneliness because it's just the two of us all day; no one to bring me a glass of water or a snack when I need one; no one to reassure me that I am doing everything I am supposed to be doing; nursing, resting, loving.

The requirements of early motherhood are actually very simple. Snuggle and nurse. Change a diaper. Take a nap. Give kisses. Feed yourself.

But no has told me that's all I need to do, and I'm convinced I am not doing enough.

And I miss my old life terribly, another reality of motherhood that no one has shared with me. I thought the love was supposed to be enough to make me forget about all that I had left behind on the other side of birth: Work and lunches with friends, evenings with my sweetie, workouts, weekend getaways, grad school research, and dreaming up new travel plans. I volunteered. I partied. I slept in. I could buy a carton of ice cream and spend the day watching movies or I could take the bus to the north shore with my buddy and spend the day climbing the cliff faces right over the ocean. In the evening, I could go to the open mic night down the street or read for hours in the bathtub. Straight up, I was an adult woman in her prime, and I could do whatever the fuck I wanted.

Now I'm at the mercy of a tiny little human who seems to think crying endlessly is the coolest way to be in the world.

And no one is telling me it's okay to miss my old life, to be frustrated by the loss of everything that had made me me up until now. No other mother has ever shared with me the paradox of feelings that come with motherhood, that the sense of loss can be just as overwhelming as the blossoming of love.

Perhaps, if someone had just acknowledged that motherhood would be as disappointing as it is fulfilling, I would have honoured the complexities of my heart rather than seeing my struggle as proof that I am not woman enough for this role.

Sometimes, in the evenings, when I'm exhausted from a day of navigating this new world, I push my baby away, begging my partner to make him stop crying so I can have just a few minutes alone in my own body without anyone touching me. Again, no one tells me this is normal, that needing time alone is okay. I feel disgusted with myself, riddled with shame. The struggle is intense, and my fear that it's just me is so strong that I don't dare share what I'm experiencing with anyone.

I feel the shame of being so much less than I am meant to be at this time in my life. Society tells me I'm supposed to love this baby phase. I was supposed to pine for it and then gratefully fall into it like it's all I've ever desired, like motherhood is the end-all, be-all of my life as a woman. That's what we get told, even though women outnumber men in universities, have access to birth control, and legislation says we're just as valuable in the work force and should be compensated equally. We get told every day by the images, stories, and sly little comments that women are made to be mothers. I am supposed to glow in this role as ultimate nurturer, creator of life.

And if I find it challenging, Pinterest holds all the secrets for how to make life organized and beautiful. Facebook is full of articles that will tell me how to get my body back and not lose myself. Instagram is the perfect place to gain inspiration from other moms who make it all look so easy.

I turn to my phone for a little bit of adult company and find myself feeling worse than before, faced with the evidence of how I fail to live up to today's expectations of mothers. My hair isn't done, my face is without makeup, showing the bags under my eyes and latest forehead pimple. My diaper bag is neither designer nor a retrofit of something way cooler. My baby wears hand-me-downs and our house is ugly as fuck. There is no tribe around us, mothers with babies on their laps, smiling for the camera. Instead I snap one more mommy-baby selfie in between the tears, finding my smile just for him and sharing it so the world, once again, assumes all is well based on a careful curation of masked moments.

But this ain't no bliss, and I stumble teary-eyed through each day.

When he's seven months old, we go on our first family camping trip. As my partner sets up the tent, I take Finley in my arms and wander down to the beautiful, wild, west-coast beach. I put him on the sand, and he starts moving. He's crawling fast enough now that I need to stay close. Sand covers his little pants so I decide to take them off. Then I decide to take off all his clothes, even his cute cloth diaper. And there's my baby, naked on the beach.

This matches my vision for what this was supposed to be. I cast aside the worries that he'll poop right there on the sand, or a bug will bite his little scrotum or, scariest of all, that someone will judge me. I just let him play. I watch him, witnessing his curiosity as he comes across seashells and pieces of driftwood. And then it washes over me, the joy. For this one little moment, I feel the joy I thought I would as a mother, and I breathe it in. Deeply. The waves crash. The air is salty on my tongue. My baby is wild and free, and my heart finds a bit of peace.

Parrish Wilson lives in rural Ontario with her two sons who are curious, insightful and love playing naked on the beach. Parrish is a mental health writer and advocate, and is currently pursuing a Masters of Arts in counselling and spirituality with a focus on menstrual health, feminist practise, and women's spirituality. You can follow her on Instagram @parrishwilson

THE FOURTH TRIMESTER

Janessa Reimer

MY HUSBAND, DUSTIN, AND I, took prenatal classes. They do a good job of preparing you for labour and birth, but no one prepared me for the fourth trimester. No one told me what might happen after the baby was born.

I remember people laughing and saying get ready to never sleep again. But I honestly had no idea just how bad it would be. It would have been so much better if those people had sat down with me, a new mom-to-be, and had a serious talk about what the lack of sleep will do to your mind, your body, and how much it truly affects you.

The lack of sleep is one thing, but combining that with having to take care of a baby that relies one you for everything? No one tells you about this.

On our first night home, I had a complete meltdown. I just couldn't get the hang of breastfeeding. I was so stressed out. My one thought was, *Well this is it, my baby is 100% going to die because I can't feed him.* I felt guilty and horrible. *Why is this so hard?* I thought. People made it look so easy. I was so grateful that Dustin went out and bought formula and figured out how to prepare it and feed our baby boy, Arden.

Breastfeeding didn't work out for me. I tried for a month or two, but I was not enjoying it. I wasn't producing enough milk, so I started pumping and supplemented with formula. I pumped for three months but it was so time consuming. By now, my mental health was really declining and the health nurse recommended that I start to slowly take out pumping sessions. The nurses in town were amazing and I truly appreciate them. It was the best decision to go with full formula feedings. Arden wasn't reliant on just me, Dustin helped out with night feedings too.

I'm not sure I have the words to describe my first week home being a new mom. There were times I wondered *what had we done?* It took me a long time to connect with Arden. I wished for my old life back. I'm an avid hiker and I love anything to do with the mountains, and I felt like I was missing out on that while caring for Arden.

I started to feel resentful toward Dustin. He didn't have to give up anything for nine months while growing a baby. He didn't have to go through the pain of giving birth or deal with the postpartum hormones and postpartum depression. I was mad that he got to go to work while I had to stay home and take care of Arden all day long without any breaks. I started to become resentful of Arden, too. He always needed me. I just couldn't get a break.

I want you to know I absolutely love my son, Arden. I don't ever regret having him. Every day I see more and more of his personality and I just fall more in love with him. But those early days were hard, and it's something we don't talk about much.

I remember one day vividly. I needed to get out of the house, so I went to visit my friend who lives an hour away. Arden was so fussy and he just wouldn't stop crying. I stayed maybe ten minutes. I was just so overwhelmed and emotional. I needed to go home. On my way home, I called Dustin saying I didn't know what to do, that Arden just wouldn't stop crying. I took Arden to the hospital, but they told me he was perfectly healthy and just a little colicky. I drove away with Arden still crying in the back seat and that's when I experienced a full-blown panic attack. I couldn't breath, and I felt dizzy. I called Dustin, and he talked me through it so that I was able to drive back to town. I dropped Arden off at his workplace and then I went home.

That evening, I couldn't touch or hold Arden. I wanted nothing to do with him. It was a terrifying feeling of not wanting anything to do with my baby. I thought there was something wrong with me. *Maybe I wasn't meant to be a mom*, I thought. I remember things got pretty dark after that. I felt like I didn't want to live anymore and that maybe everyone would be better off without me. Even reliving that moment now is so heartbreaking. I remember that darkness vividly.

I mourned my old life. Everyone asked about the baby but not very many people asked me how I was doing. If they did ask, they didn't want to hear anything negative. I began to feel like no one truly cared about me. I felt so alone and guilty about everything. I felt selfish for longing for the life we had before Arden came along. I missed the time I used to spend with Dustin without the addition of this little person who required so much. I didn't want to just suck it up and give up all the things that Dustin and I did together before Arden. I wanted Arden to join our lives.

I reached out for help. I was so grateful that I had the best nurses looking after me. I saw a counsellor, and I started going on short hikes and hanging out with friends. But even with all that, I just could not stop feeling so depressed. I went on antidepressants. I felt like a failure at first and went on and off them for a while. Back on the medication, I finally woke up one morning and just felt happy.

New moms, you're not alone. No one should be ashamed of going through postpartum depression and anxiety. It is more common than you know.

Janessa Reimer is mom to Arden and lives in Claresholm, Alberta. She is a certified postpartum doula, helping parents with the transition of bringing a newborn home. You can find her on Facebook and Instagram @serenitymaternalsupport

WHAT IS PERINATAL MENTAL HEALTH?

Dr. Simone Vigod

THE WORLD HEALTH ORGANIZATION TALKS about the importance of conceptualizing health as much more than simply the absence of illness. Specifically, in the preamble to their constitution, they state*:

- Health is a state of complete physical, mental and social well-being and not merely the absence of disease or infirmity.
- The enjoyment of the highest attainable standard of health is one of the fundamental rights of every human being without distinction of race, religion, political belief, economic or social condition.

As such, perinatal mental health can be thought of as a state of being where a person and their family are experiencing more than the absence of depression, anxiety, or other psychiatric symptoms. Ideally, it means that a perinatal person and their family are able to experience this stage of life in a state of overall well-being, and that every person and family has a right to achieve this. My belief is that it is crucial to address a multitude of intersecting social and clinical factors, on both individual and systemic levels, to promote mental health in the perinatal period.

The Diagnostic and Statistical Manual of Mental Disorders (DSM) version 5, the manual used in North America that outlines the diagnostic criteria for diagnosable psychiatric disorders, allows for a diagnosis of a depressive episode to include the specifier "with peripartum onset" when symptoms of depression have begun either in pregnancy or within the first four weeks postpartum. In the International Classification of Diseases version 11 (ICD-11), a diagnosis of "mental disorders associated with pregnancy, childbirth or the puerperium) is considered if a syndrome of any mental health symptomatology develops in pregnancy or within about six weeks postpartum. This diagnosis can be given alongside any diagnosis of a mental disorder, including depression or any other psychiatric condition.

The requirement from the DSM-5 and ICD-11 diagnostic categorizations that symptoms must start in pregnancy or in the first four to six weeks postpartum comes from research that suggests that if there is a biological mechanism that distinguishes "perinatal" mental illness from mental illnesses occurring outside the "perinatal period", that biological mechanism is probably hormone-related and most likely to be responsible for the conditions that arise at this stage. In contrast, it is thought that when symptoms of mental illness arise prior to pregnancy, or later in the postpartum period, the mechanisms that underlie their development are probably more similar to those that underlie the development of mental illness at any life stage, including biological, psychological, and social factors.

That being said, when thinking about how to achieve perinatal mental "health" (as opposed to only the absence of illness), people with lived experience and experts who have worked with patients and conducted research for many years, tend to imagine the "perinatal period" a bit more broadly—both in terms of when the perinatal period starts, and when it ends.

There is an emerging focus on conceptualizing the "perinatal period" as starting in the time before pregnancy, when individuals and their families are planning a pregnancy. This is because prior mental illness - especially when untreated or undertreated—is one of the strongest risk factors for mental illness in pregnancy and postpartum, and also because of the very specific issues that come up around decisions regarding use of psychiatric medications in pregnancy and in breastfeeding. In the "preconception," there is an opportunity to ensure that pre-existing conditions are optimally managed, in order to prevent the relapse of these conditions around the time of pregnancy. Many pregnancies are unplanned, so this is not always possible, but when it is, this can be a very useful approach.

Similarly, there is a strong argument for mental illness that arises after six weeks postpartum and up to about one year postpartum to also be considered "perinatal." This is because unique issues in the transition to parenthood that can affect mental health—lack of sleep, social isolation, constant caregiving of an infant, parental identity, re-negotiation of roles with intimate partners, among others—occur to varying degrees throughout the first year postpartum. When planning supports and treatment services, it makes sense to include those who have these similar or shared psychological experiences—and not to exclude people simply because their symptoms did not develop in the first four to six weeks postpartum. While many similar issues extend beyond the first year postpartum, when infants become toddlers this can necessitate different approaches to treatment, especially with regard to parenting.

More than postpartum depression

Any mental health condition can recur or develop anew during the perinatal period. The most common conditions are depression, anxiety disorders like generalized anxiety disorder and panic disorder, stressor-related disorders such as post-traumatic stress disorder, and obsessive-compulsive disorders. One may also see alcohol or substance use disorders, or eating disorders, among others. More rarely, conditions such as mania or psychosis that suggest the development of bipolar disorder, as well as schizophrenia are observed.

What is unique to the perinatal period is often the way in which symptoms of these conditions are experienced. For example, the main symptoms of depression are sadness and anhedonia, which means loss of interest or pleasure. These symptoms are accompanied by additional symptoms such as difficulty with sleep, concentration and appetite, feeling or seeming "slowed down" or "keyed up," as well as by negative thoughts such as guilt and worthlessness, or suicidal ideation. In the perinatal period, people may have difficulty sleeping specifically because they are worried that something terrible will happen to their baby while they sleep. Specific negative thoughts might include feeling that one is failing as a parent, or guilt about not being able to (or wanting to) establish breastfeeding.

Anxiety

Anxiety is also common in the perinatal period. Often, the anxious thoughts revolve around health and safety of the person, their baby and/or family; worries may also centre around partner relationships and financial issues where there are unique impacts of a pregnancy and having a newborn. While many new and expectant parents will worry, sometimes the anxiety becomes very severe and/or hard to control. This can mean that there is a mental health condition that would benefit from treatment.

Anxiety can be present in perinatal depression, and anxiety disorders can be diagnosed in addition to or instead of depression. For example, generalized anxiety disorder is an anxiety disorder characterized by excessive anxiety and worry about a number of things for six months or more that is accompanied by physical symptoms such as tension and irritability. Panic disorder is an anxiety disorder where attacks of panic seem to come out of the blue, and people live in fear of having another one. Sometimes this can result in people being afraid of going out of the house, and/or to crowded places, a symptom that could be very isolating for a new parent. Social anxiety disorder, where people feel very anxious around being exposed to scrutiny by others, can be very difficult in the perinatal period—when people are already often feeling insecure about what they say and do.

OCD and Intrusive Thoughts

It is also fairly common perinatally for people to experience recurrent intrusive thoughts or images of something terrible happening, including thoughts or images of they, themselves doing something to harm their baby. Often these latter thoughts and images are very distressing and people feel ashamed of them, even though they know that they would never intentionally harm their baby. For some, these thoughts are fleeting, and do not occur with a specific mental health issue—other times they are part of the symptoms experienced in perinatal depression. Obsessive-compulsive disorder, or OCD, may be diagnosed when these recurrent intrusive thoughts are causing marked anxiety and distress, and/or when repetitive acts that temporarily reduce the anxiety around the thoughts—like checking on the baby repeatedly due to thoughts that the baby will stop breathing—are so time-consuming as to result in impairment in social, occupational or other important areas of functioning.

PTSD

The diagnosis of "post-traumatic stress disorder" is being discussed more and more in relation to the perinatal period. Those with pre-existing, post-traumatic stress disorder may see their symptoms worsen in pregnancy, labour and after delivery. Others may report new-onset nightmares, flashbacks and other feelings of distress related to their birth experience. For some, the impacts of such experiences may improve on their own over time, with reassurance. However, people whose symptoms are ongoing, and who begin to develop ongoing difficulty, especially around being able to experience positive emotions around their child or about being a parent, may need additional treatment.

Bipolar and Psychosis

While the above conditions are the ones that people most commonly experience, there are more rare and acutely severe forms of mental illness that are seen in the perinatal period, such as postpartum psychosis. Postpartum psychosis—affecting less than one in 1000 women or childbearing individuals—most commonly occurs in the early days and weeks after childbirth, often among those who have prior diagnoses of bipolar disorder or who go on to develop bipolar disorder. Symptoms of postpartum psychosis may include appearing confused, developing false beliefs about oneself, one's baby or others, or hearing voices or noises that are not really there. Postpartum psychosis can become a safety issue if a person's false beliefs lead them to think that they should harm themselves or their child. For safety reasons, a suspected postpartum psychosis should be considered a medical emergency. If a new parent is psychotic, they should not be left alone on their own, or with their baby, but should be brought to an emergency department for assessment, possible hospital admission and medical treatment.

Evidence-based treatment for perinatal mental illness

For almost any set of mental health symptoms to be diagnosed as a psychiatric condition or disorder, the symptoms usually must be present on more days than not for a specific length of time, and must cause significant distress for the person experiencing them, or cause impairment in social, occupational or other areas of functioning. When a person doesn't meet these criteria, they may still benefit from support, but probably would not be diagnosed with a mental illness or require medical treatment. All those who are pregnant and postpartum, whether they have a diagnosable mental health condition or not, may benefit from practical and emotional social support, healthy eating, exercise and adequate sleep. Attention to factors that might be worsening mental health symptoms are really important, especially serious problems such as substance abuse or domestic or intimate partner violence.

When a person has been diagnosed with one of the more common mental health conditions, such as perinatal depression or anxiety, generally, a "stepped care model" of treatment is recommended. In a stepped care model, the most effective and least intensive treatment(s) for a condition are tried first, followed by more intensive treatments when needed. For example, for mild symptoms of postpartum depression, there is evidence that psychosocial treatments such as peer support (e.g. parent-to-parent support) or supportive counselling from a health care provider, either on a 1:1 basis or in a group can be helpful on their own.

There is also evidence for the effectiveness of guided self-help, Internet or paper-based self-guided interventions that might include assistance from a trained coach. When psychosocial strategies do not result in an improvement or symptoms, or when the initial symptoms are more severe, formal psychological therapy delivered by a trained mental health professional is recommended. The most well-studied types of therapy are Cognitive Behaviour Therapy (CBT) for all types of illnesses and Interpersonal Therapy (IPT) for postpartum depression specifically. Other therapies such as Behavioural Activation (BA) are also showing good effectiveness for perinatal depression and anxiety.

Medication

When therapy on its own is not sufficient to improve symptoms, or when symptoms are severe, medications should be considered. Medications may also be considered in the setting of milder symptoms when an individual has previously responded to medication or prefers medication treatment to therapy. For perinatal depression, anxiety, OCD and PTSD, antidepressant medications are usually the first type of medication considered. Other types of medication may be added or used instead of these, for example when people are having difficulty sleeping or when antidepressant medication is insufficient to control the symptoms. The decision to use medication always involves balancing the potential benefits of the medication with any potential risks, including side effects as well as the safety of medication exposure to a fetus or infant. Most antidepressant medications are considered to have relatively few risks in pregnancy or lactation. Medication may be especially important for those who are suffering greatly from psychiatric symptoms that may themselves have a negative impact on the developing fetus or child. The decision about when and if to start medication is a personal and individualized one that should be discussed with a doctor.

Those with conditions such as bipolar disorder and psychosis will benefit from a comprehensive consultation with a physician about the most appropriate medication and psychotherapy treatments for their conditions. As indicated, postpartum psychosis is a medical emergency, almost always requiring a period of hospitalization and medication for stabilization and treatment.

How long does perinatal mental illness last?

Without treatment—or with not enough treatment—a perinatal mental illness can become chronic. Sometimes symptoms may improve on their own over months to years. However, when a condition becomes chronic, this means it continues indefinitely either with ongoing symptoms, or becomes relapsing and remitting (i.e. an episode occurs and then goes away, but comes back again at a later time).

The causes of all mental illnesses are complex, and involve an array of intersecting biological, psychological and social factors. Specific to perinatal mental illness, and where most of the research to date is in women, we know that having a personal or family history of any mental illness is a risk factor, as is having a previous mental illness. Biologically, some people's brains may be sensitive to the hormonal fluctuations that occur with pregnancy and after delivery, and that triggers a mental health syndrome even in the absence of a history of mental illness or other risk factors. Psychosocial risk factors that greatly increase the chances that someone will develop perinatal depression include poor social support, and major stressors that range from job loss to a sick child to domestic or intimate partner violence. However, none of these risk factors mean that a person will definitely develop a postpartum mental illness, and some will develop perinatal mental illness with no risk factors at all.

What to do if you need help

I think that the most important piece to remember is that perinatal mental illnesses are treatable. So, it is essential to create hope for people and open the door so people get the right type of care. A person whose partner or loved one is suffering can help by providing validation - that perinatal mental illness is real, common, that it is not a person's fault that they have developed it and that having this illness does not mean that they are a bad parent. Further, a person should never be made to feel that they are not getting better because "they are not trying hard enough". Treatment may take time and may require trying various treatment options alone or in combination, so it is important to reassure someone that although the road to recovery may feel slow, they can indeed recover.

There are many ways to receive help. Postpartum Support International (www.postpartum.net) provides peer support and information about counselling services all around the world. People can also be open with their health care providers (e.g. midwives, nurses, primary care providers, obstetricians) about how they are feeling. The health care provider can help to determine what type of care is needed and how to arrange it.

Dr. Simone Vigod is the Head of the Department of Psychiatry at Women's College Hospital in Toronto, Ontario, where she practices as a psychiatrist in the Reproductive Life Stages program at that provides care to women with mental health issues across their reproductive life cycle from menstruation to menopause. She is a leading expert in perinatal mood disorders and has conducted some of the largest studies worldwide on maternal mental illness around the time of pregnancy. Connect with Dr. Vigod on Twitter @simonevigod

POST-ADOPTION DEPRESSION

Erin Paterson

I WALK UP THE FRONT steps of my house with my seven-week-old daughter nestled in the crook of my arm. After pushing the door open, I quickly kick off my shoes and place my baby on a yellow checkered blanket on the living room floor. Once she is safely settled, I close the blinds on the front windows, blocking out the beautiful summer day.

I want to be invisible to the world. It's in the safety of my home, away from the gaze of others, that my emotions are set free. A guttural wail emerges from my throat and tears spring from my eyes. I pick my baby up off the floor and press her gently to my shuddering chest. My arms wrap around her tiny body, protecting her. I need to hold her tight, to feel her body against my own, to know that I am her mom.

My husband and I adopted our daughter. We brought her home when she was just ten days old. For the first month, we lived with the constant threat of having to give her back. We knew there was a chance after spending weeks bonding with her and falling in love with her that our daughter's birth mother might change her mind.

We had just passed that waiting period and felt relieved, but we had many hurdles ahead of us before we would legally be considered her parents—more visits from the social worker, a final report to the government, and a court date when the adoption would hopefully be finalized. At any point during the process, our suitability as parents could be called into question. Even though the chances were slim, I feared our baby could still be taken away from us.

It wasn't just the pressures from adoption that were getting to me. I was struggling with a range of conflicting emotions resulting from a long journey through infertility. That's why I was unexpectedly set off by a stranger in line at the coffee shop before rushing home to wail in the darkness.

"Congratulations," the stranger says, motioning to the stroller.

"Thank you," I say, smiling back at her as we shuffle a few steps closer to the cashier.

"Can I look at your baby?" she asks.

"Sure" I say, pulling the sunshade back to reveal my sleeping daughter and her pudgy round face, the tuft of reddish hair on the top of her head, and her incredibly long eyelashes resting against her cheeks.

"She's so beautiful," she says.

"Thank you," I say back, smiling with the pride of a new mom.

"She looks just like you."

And there it is. Her comment feels like a stab to my heart. It isn't the first time someone says that to me. I guess it is just a natural thing people do but these types of comparisons serve to remind me of my inability to conceive. Normally, I just smile and nod but I am so sick of people comparing my baby's features to my own that I blurt out: "No she doesn't, because she's adopted."

"Oh wow, that's so wonderful!" she says, reaching over and placing a sympathetic hand on my shoulder.

"Well she still looks like you anyways dear. No one would ever know. It's the same as having a baby because you got her so young. She will never know the difference."

I can't get out of the coffee shop fast enough. I am annoyed that people have such a narrow view of how families are created. Her comments rub my infertility in my face, poking at that sore spot that told me I was different from everyone else, that made me feel inadequate. So I rush home, close the blinds and sit in the darkness of my home, crying and holding my baby, away from any hurtful comments.

The thing that I didn't realize at the time was that I was still grieving the loss of my fertility. Adopting a baby had fulfilled my need to be a parent, but I was still infertile. The feelings that went along with those struggles didn't go away just because I had become a mom. "You must be happy now," close friends and family would say. "Of course," I'd reply. But even though my dreams had come true, I was also desperately sad. It had taken us five-and-a-half-years to have a child.

We had started out like most couples trying to conceive naturally and not expecting any problems. Twelve months later, we found ourselves under the care of a fertility doctor. We spent countless early mornings at the fertility clinic getting blood tests and ultrasounds and waiting to meet with the doctor, having test after test after test, the results of which were all inconclusive. We tried each fertility protocol two or three times before moving on to the next option, which eventually led to two failed in-vitro fertilizations.

I had a row of bruises running along my stomach from all the self-administered needles of fertility medication. I had gained ten pounds and was suffering from depression. Month after month, there was a phone call from the clinic nurse telling me that I wasn't pregnant. Worst of all, though, was the loss of hope that came with knowing that my body had failed us again. My husband and I spent some time getting second opinions and investigating other options like donor egg, surrogacy and child free living. Eventually we decided to try adoption.

To become *adopt ready*, we had to go through parenting classes, be interviewed by a social worker five times, submit our finances and have a medical checkup done. There is no centralized waiting list when you are adopting privately, so we had to register individually with adoption lawyers across the country. Miraculously, a year-and-a-half after starting the process of adoption, we were chosen by a birth mother to be the parents of her baby.

I had no idea what it meant to be an adoptive mom. In the early days, I wondered if the love I felt for my daughter was the same love as other parents felt for their biological children. When my daughter cried and it didn't freak me out like other moms, I worried there was something wrong with me. *Was I missing that maternal bond to my child? Would my daughter reject me as her mom?* I was concerned she might have health problems because I wasn't able to breastfeed her. I was terrified that when I went back to work she would forget who I was. On top of that, we were still living with the threat of her being taken away from us. It wasn't until she was 11 months old that our approval came through and we were officially declared her legal parents.

Raising an adopted child was different in many ways from natural conception. As a new mom, there were so many factors impacting my mental health. I knew about postpartum depression, but I dismissed my feelings because I had not given birth to my child. Besides, everyone else expected me to be happy. So I struggled to come to terms with all the fearful thoughts in my head, much of the time on my own. It wouldn't be until years later, my daughter, a preschooler by then, that I learned about post-adoption depression and it clicked. *Oh my gosh, that's what happened to me*, I thought. It was then that I was finally able to acknowledge that indeed my feelings were valid even if no one else understood them at the time.

I learned that post-adoption depression, or PADS for short, affects up to 32% of adoptive parents and involves many of the same symptoms as postpartum depression and anxiety. Treatment can involve therapy and/or medication and a good place to start is with your family doctor.

*https://static1.squarespace.com/static/531227d8e4b04bcb37e61666/t/59d50e6df14aa17707cca16a/1507135086853/PADS+Tipsheet.pdf

I think it is important to share my struggles so that others can understand what it is like to experience infertility and post-adoption depression. More importantly, though, I hope that sharing my story will help someone else who is going through a similar experience.

Erin Paterson is mom to Emma and lives in Toronto. She is positively impacting people's lives by sharing her stories about infertility, genetic testing, and adoption through writing and public speaking. You can find Erin on Instagram @erinpaterson_allgoodthings or visit her website at erinpaterson.com

A STRANGER IN THE HOUSE

Tara Mandarano

IT'S AMAZING WHAT A SECOND glance at first-time motherhood reveals. Those early days are steeped so strongly in my memory. Before my daughter was born, my brain drew up a blueprint of what I thought life would be like, post-baby. It included nursing in the rocking chair in the middle of the night, endless cute outfits, and an overall sense of cozy, snowed-in bliss.

I didn't count on having a panic attack about which onesie to pack in my hospital bag, like it was the most crucial decision I'd ever make. I couldn't know that I would struggle with breastfeeding no matter where I sat, that the cheerful Hooter Hider cover-ups would go unworn.

But the part that caught me off guard the most was the sheer time of year—winter, the most beastly season to have a baby. It was not cozy; it was confining. It was not blissful; it was bleak. I remember staring zombie-like at daytime TV while my daughter took short naps. She was learning the difference between day and night, and I was just trying not to fall apart.

I remember the profound relief of escaping to the bathroom, alone, closing the door on my new reality and greedily grabbing a few minutes for myself. How a five-minute shower felt like a vacation. On the days when it was possible, it was my salvation.

My original sketch of our family life was woefully incomplete, but there was no way to know what lay ahead without living it. Going through it. All I heard from new parents was how "in love" with their baby they were. This constant stream of rose-coloured language left me feeling lacking when it was my turn.

Sure, I was amazed at this tiny being before me, and I loved her with a fierceness I never would have fathomed, but I was also totally terrified, sleep deprived, and nearly manic with all the mayhem a new child brings.

I remember the anticlimactic feeling once the baby was born and everyone went home.

Looking at that tiny, unfamiliar face and not recognizing the reality of the child in my arms. The possibilities of the dream child gone, the actual baby a monumental mystery.

I recollect how a friend put it: that it was strange to have a stranger in the house.

I remember the sum of all the things I didn't know about parenthood crushing down on me, the pressure to get everything perfect. I recall putting my relationship on the back burner and forgetting to check how it was doing. How my hubby and I went from lovebirds to squabblers in the span of weeks.

It's astonishing how much your brain blocks out over time. It's only when you're around another newborn that the unsavoury stuff you've shoved in a mental drawer comes crashing open. The advent of the poonamis. Heavy-duty painkillers. Stool softeners. The endless patting, swaddling, walking, rocking. The sheer terror involved in giving a newborn a bath.

I remember obsessively watching the clock for the next scheduled feeding. Trying to figure out formula doses, the albatross of breast pumps. Not realizing the true purpose and brilliance of a onesie's design until well after the fact.

My only solace was a postnatal support group held every week. As mothers of newborns and toddlers, we could share our struggles with postpartum anxiety and depression and not feel shamed. We could take turns and talk, and not have our thoughts and feelings carelessly shoved under the "baby blues" label. For me, it was a safe place to tell my story and see myself reflected in other mothers' realities. What a difference validation makes.

As time went on, things got better, and I discovered that rocking chairs were the perfect place to read my daughter board books. I realized that she could sleep in the same thing she wore during the day and nobody would notice. I learned that there is a certain kind of wonder to be found in winter. Through her fresh eyes, I saw how a blizzard could be considered beautiful again, when it's the first one you've ever seen.

Now I'm able to look back and relive all the wondrous moments, too. The day she discovered her arm was actually attached to her body. The way she liked to sleep all snuggled up on our chests. The sound of her first giggle in the bathtub.

I can admit now that I was only half in love with her then. I was still getting to know her, bit by bit. Today I am head over heels, and there is a deluge of happiness in my heart.

My life is not always easier with her in it, but it is infinitely better for it.

Today I am two years past this experience, and I'm still writing my way out of it. There were a lot of dark moments those first few months of figuring out what to do and how to feel, but I'd do them all again to have the beautiful blessing that is my daughter.

Tara Mandarano is mom to a seven-year-old-daughter. She is also a Best-of-the-Net-nominated writer. Her work is featured in the anthology *BIG: Stories About Life in Plus-Sized Bodies*, and she has also been published in *The Washington Post, HuffPost, Motherwell*, and *Today's Parent*. You can follow her on Instagram and Twitter @taramandarano.

BRAIN OFFLINE

Dr. Walker Ladd

It is surreal to know the brain has shut down. Like a cutting of permanent wires, my brain was offline.

Around six weeks postpartum, Ziggy started sleeping through the night. I did not. When he slept on my chest, my mind raced. I would slide him over to my husband and try to sleep on the living room floor. But I was still awake. I stayed awake for the next three weeks.

My primary care provider told me to drink milk at night. I stayed awake. She told me to take 50 mg of Benadryl. I stayed awake. At my six-week checkup, she prescribed Paxil. I had a horrible reaction to it and stayed awake.

One of the strongest memories of my postpartum depression and anxiety is that I believed I had lost my ability to sleep. The cycle of anxiety began in the early evening and would become a night of panic attacks. I thought Ziggy would be better off without me.

No sleep. One week, two weeks, three weeks. I started spending the night on the living room floor. Night after night on that floor. When I heard Ziggy wake up, I went in and fed him, then headed back out to the living room floor where I didn't sleep.

One night, around Christmas, I decided it would never end, that I would never be able to sleep, that my precious son didn't deserve to have such a defective mother and that I should jump off of the Aurora Bridge near our house. I had already contemplated suicide many times by then but had not attempted it. But that night, as a marathon of the movie *A Christmas Story* played over and over, I wanted my life to end.

I got in my car. We didn't live that far from the bridge. It was so dark that night. And icy. I kept trying to figure out how I could stop on the side of the road and jump without hurting the drivers in the cars behind me. It was not their fault I wanted to die.

In the Queen Anne neighborhood of Seattle, there is an on-ramp that comes off of a curvy residential street. I drove onto the bridge and put my hazards on. I wanted it over so badly. I kept driving to the other side of the bridge, circling around, and trying it again. I never stopped. I eventually drove home and got back on the living room floor. No one ever knew I had left. I said nothing the next day. The thoughts of suicide were constant. I thought about the times my own father attempted suicide and failed and was ashamed that I was like him—having gone that far in trying but failing.

Later the next day, I was standing behind my husband who was changing Ziggy's diapers, when I passed out from exhaustion. Throughout my postpartum depression and anxiety, my husband kept telling me that it was all under my control. *Just change your mind*, was his mantra. At the time, he meant that he believed I could stop suffering through my own volition. By just changing my mind. The implication was that it was all in my head metaphorically and that I was failing at fixing it. He didn't understand, not sure he does to this day, and I don't blame him. What he didn't know was that my mind, the organic brain matter inside of my skull—the negative space between synapses definitely needed changing through medical intervention. He was suffering his own battle with anxiety and fear. He has since shared with me that my passing out that day was as scared as he had ever been.

Nonetheless, the message I got from him was that these physical symptoms were the result of my personal choice. In other words, if I fixed my own thinking, I would suddenly sleep like a baby and be hungry and happy and not want to drive to the highest bridge in Seattle and jump. This is why I didn't tell him about my driving to the Aurora Bridge when I got home that night. He wouldn't know what to do other than tell me to do something myself. I needed someone's help, not more pressure to fix myself. He wouldn't be a soft place to fall that night, nor any night to come.

From my station on the living room floor, I called my internship supervisor and told her I was suicidal. While she had no experience with perinatal mood or anxiety disorders and no references to share, she did say something that shook me to my core. *Walker, if you kill yourself, Ziggy will never be okay. Ever.* I knew she was right.

I looked through my clinical textbooks from my graduate studies and clinical training. Two books became professional lifelines to recovery. The first, Shaila Misri's (1991) book, *Shouldn't I be happy: Emotional problems of pregnant and postpartum women*, had been assigned in my life cycle course. After speaking with my supervisor that night, I scoured that book and tried to track down the phone number for Dr. Shaila Misri in Vancouver, British Columbia, and I left a long voicemail message asking for help. The next day, surprised that she called me back, I spoke with her on the phone, and she assured me that I could be successfully treated with the right medication. She shared, *You can't compete with chemistry,* and connected me with a psychiatric nurse practitioner in Seattle. I left a voice message for the nurse practitioner, who called me back and did a short intake over the phone. She told me to either self-admit to the hospital for suicidal ideation or have someone with me 24 hours a day until I was stabilized on medication, and then she booked my appointment.

I went to see the nurse practitioner who took one look at me and got samples out of her private stash for me to take home. She wrote a prescription for antidepressants and that night, I slept for the first time in three weeks.

I continued to get better. My recovery was slow, but it was a recovery.

When I got pregnant with my beautiful daughter, Miles, two years later, I was referred to an excellent obstetrician and a great therapist familiar with perinatal mental health. I had a happy pregnancy, birth, and postpartum period with my sweet baby girl, Miles. I was symptom-free, even though my obstetrician had to tell me to bring my own antidepressants from home so that the nurses wouldn't bother me about taking it while breastfeeding. We did it, my girl and me. We did it. The four days I spent in the hospital with Miles was possibly the happiest I have ever been, even to this day.

Dr. Walker Ladd has been a thought leader in the field of maternal mental health for nearly two decades. Her book, *Transformed by Postpartum Depression: Women's stories of trauma and growth* (Praeclarus, 2020), was based on her grounded theory study of the traumatic and nature of untreated perinatal mood and anxiety disorders, and subsequent posttraumatic growth for 25 women. You can find Walker on Instagram @dralkerladd and her website is www.walkerladd.com

WHAT'S REALLY GOING ON?

Olivia Scobie

I WAS YOUNGER THAN MOST when I became a parent. I didn't really know anything about babies, other than I thought they were cute, which was a significant factor in my decision to keep the baby (that decision-making seems laughable now).

When I was pregnant, I had a vague vision about what life with a baby would look like that was mostly anchored in the idea of long stroller-walks with coffee or holding a sleepy baby while I chatted with friends. Even though I was nervous about being a solo parent without an income, I wasn't scared in any significant way.

Younger me had the kind of hopeful optimism that only youth can provide, which is hard to distinguish from foolishness.

Life with an actual baby, instead of the fantasy in my head, was a shock. The birth was long and traumatic, the baby was born with several medical issues, and figuring out how to feed a baby was a nightmare. The baby did not sleep the way it had been described in pregnancy books, and instead fell into a cycle of waking and crying for 40 minutes and then sleeping on me for 40 minutes. I hadn't even had time to recover from the birth before I found myself weary to the bone and felt myself slipping into a deep depression. I cried a lot, as I was pretty sure I had ruined my life.

Time passed so slowly, and I remember looking at the clock throughout the day, hoping at least an hour had passed, only to realize it had only been about 20 minutes. I felt like a failure at mothering and couldn't imagine feeling joy again, and soon found that my only comfort was in the last few moments as I was drifting off to sleep, when I imagined that my body would give out from the exhaustion and simply not wake up.

Because I was young and single and poor, it didn't feel particularly safe to tell anyone how I was feeling. I was afraid that they would take my baby, or worse, confirm all my fears that I was a terrible mother and the baby deserved better. When medical professionals tried to check in with me, I'd lie and say everything was fine. I got really good at performing good parenting when I had to, but also knew I had to do something to help myself.

When the baby was two months old, I decided to go back to school, which may seem like an unusual way to treat depression, but it gave me the lifeline I needed to survive. Although I didn't feel better for a long time, taking breaks from the baby gave me the ability to rest my nervous system and connect to the non-parent parts of me.

It took me several years before I thought I could have another baby. By now, I was partnered and more financially secure, so even though I was scared, I hoped that everything would be different because my life circumstances were so different.

It was different the second time, but not in the way I was anticipating. My feelings of depression were less intense, but I was overcome with perinatal anxiety. It started in pregnancy, and the racing thoughts and buzzing in my body felt impossible to turn off. It wasn't helping that when the baby was born, they had jaundice so severe they had to be hospitalized. I was flooded with intrusive thoughts of the baby dying, so much so that I could hardly sleep, even though this baby gave me long chunks to rest. I was angry and panicked and overwhelmed throughout the days and felt like I was alienating everyone around me. I suffered like this for months, until my family doctor checked in with me at a well-baby visit. When she asked how I was doing, and I mumbled my usual, *fine, just tired phrase*, she called me out.

"I know you. I know you're not okay. What's really going on?" she probed.

I crumbled. And cried. And by the end of that visit I had a prescription for anti-depressants and a referral for both group and individual therapy. Within weeks, I felt like I could cope again, and the ability to talk about my feelings gave me incredible relief. I can't say that I ever felt great during my maternity leave, because truthfully, I just didn't enjoy being a stay-at-home mom. I found it boring and exhausting and incredibly loud. But I was able to manage until my second baby was nine months, when I returned to school again.

I love being in school and am happiest as a student, but being in school was also a form of therapy for me. Studying the sociology of gender, families, and mothering gave me language to understand what was happening to me, and that my personal narrative was part of a larger narrative about the under supporting of parents and the exhaustive nature of care work. I became fascinated with the relationship between the culture of parenting and the impact it has on maternal identity development. *Does anyone feel like a good mom? Who is seen as a good mom by their community members—and who isn't? Why do moms feel so guilty all the time?* I wanted to answer it all!

Like so many postpartum depression and anxiety survivors, I was so shaped by my experience that I wanted to help parents in similar situations, so I left a job in adult education to become a social worker. I now support parents full time. I have a private social work practice where I offer perinatal counselling, run a not-for-profit that offers free services to parents in Toronto, Ontario, as well as train other professionals how to provide care for parents having a difficult time adjusting to life with a baby.

I was asked recently if I would go through postpartum depression and anxiety all over again if it meant it would lead me here. This stumped me. I love what I do, but postpartum depression and anxiety robbed me of a lot. It's always unbelievable to me when I meet people who enjoy the postpartum experience, and it fills me with grief that I'll never get to experience that. I can't say that I would do it again if I had the choice, but I do feel grateful that I was able to make such a difficult experience meaningful and I've found a lot of healing in being able to offer parents who are in it the type of support I wish I had had the first time.

Olivia Scobie is a mom of two and lives in Toronto, Ontario. She is a queer social worker who specializes in perinatal mood, birth and reproductive trauma, and perinatal loss. She is also the author of *Impossible Parenting: Creating A New Culture Of Mental Health For Parents*. You can find Olivia on Instagram @oliviasunwantedparentingadvice

BLACK HOLE

Lisa Molinelli

My birth plan went out the window.

I am standing in my hospital room, looking out at the blackness of the winter night. It is 2:30 in the morning, two nights after I had my baby via emergency C-section. I can't breathe. My heart is pounding, and my entire body is on fire. I am terrified and feel alarmingly unsafe and panicked. Asleep on the guest cot is my mother, but I find no solace in that. My husband has gone home to sleep and I desperately want him to be here. I don't know how long I have been in this state and only dimly recall going back to bed.

This is just the beginning of my journey into a black hole of deep despair. The next night my husband pulls into our driveway with our tiny new bundle of baby boy. I gaze at him and I say, "We are finally home." I swear he smiles a big beautiful smile back. I think that arriving home will be what I need to quell the growing anxiety inside me. We almost didn't make it out of the hospital because our son's weight dropped. I had tons of colostrum, and I insisted on breastfeeding so the nurses attached a tube to my breast to try to get his weight up. It wasn't fun and now the pain medication from the C-section has worn off.

I am 40 years old, and our son is an in-vitro fertilization baby. I was considered a high-risk pregnancy, and if I didn't go into the hospital twice a week for non-stress tests, I wouldn't have known that he was in distress the morning before his due date. I felt some low back pain but that was all. It turned out that my cervix was sealed shut. I found that ironic because I spent my pregnancy worried that it was too open. I had had surgery years previous to remove scar tissue from a cervical surgery I had in my twenties. The nurse then had said that I had to be careful when I got pregnant and that stayed in my mind. The doctor then tried to open my cervix to no avail and he informed me that I would have to have a C-section right away.

I called my husband who was working in the city and told him he needed to come to the hospital right away. I was in shock and stayed that way for the entire labour and birth procedure. I had a really easy pregnancy. Not even morning sickness plagued me. It was a blessing compared to the eight years of trying to get pregnant.

Now we are home, and I am relieved. But that lasts a nanosecond. As soon as I walk through the door, I am hit with an unbearable wave of fear and panic. The walls close in on me, my body burns hot then cold, my heart pounds and my stomach twists in sickening fear. I am consumed by panic. I move from room to room throughout the house trying to find something familiar, something that makes me feel safe. I find nothing. The world has turned grey and cold with sharp edges. I can't recall my life before baby.

My mind is reeling, searching wildly to find my identity, the me before the baby. The *I* of who I am, who I was, is gone. Forever. It feels like I am seeing out of the eyes of a stranger. This is not my life. Nothing is familiar. I find no solace in my home. I feel that I have just lost my life in a blink of an eye. It's as if the me that existed for 40 years has never actually existed at all.

How can I explain this feeling of loss? I can't even rationalize why I'm reacting this way. I can't articulate it well and I certainly can't share any of this with my husband or my mother.

The next day arrives, and rock-hard breasts have me running to the shower to relieve the pain. In the shower, alone, I break down into guttural wails that seem to come from the depths of my soul. I am in acute agony. I beg the powers that be to free me from this hell. I don't want this. I feel trapped beyond belief and there is no escape. My sobbing is so loud, my husband and mother rush up the stairs to see what is going on. My mother knows then that something is wrong. My husband does not.

Over the next month, I try my best to repress my anxiety and fight against what I'm feeling. At this time, I do not know what postpartum mood disorders are. I only know of the possible, two-week baby blues period. Surely, I affirm, I can fix this on my own. My mind is determined to win this battle, and I successfully rebel in my denial. After all, I have tons of knowledge on mind power and the ability to shift perceptions and see things differently. I know about neuroplasticity. I can do this!

I am wrong. One month postpartum, I stop breastfeeding after developing a bladder infection and going on medication. I was so hypervigilant about making sure my son got enough breast milk, and it was pushing me farther over the edge. Now I'm not breastfeeding him at all, and I feel like a failure. I can't eat and I can't sleep. My mother is pleading with me to get help; I keep refusing and then the scary thoughts begin.

I am plagued by nightmares while I am awake. My panic attacks appear out of nowhere. I feel haunted by an invisible force. I am in a constant state of anxiety, and I am terrified that I am crazy. I am also afraid to go on medication for perinatal mental illness for what it might do to my body, but I'm more terrified I'll go crazy if I don't get help. My mom and I google "postpartum depression" and we find Brooke Shields' book, *Down Came the Rain: My Journey Through Postpartum Depression*. I download and read it and it's the first feeling of relief I have since my son was born. Her story is similar to mine. I feel a glimmer of hope. It's time to surrender and get help.

My mom and I contact my family doctor. He writes a prescription for an antidepressant, but I soon learn that I'm not out of my nightmare just yet. I am in an acute state of postpartum anxiety and depression, and it takes a few weeks for the medication to work. I still can't sleep and after reading about postpartum mood disorders online, I am now terrified that I may hurt my baby. I am a hypervigilant, A-type personality. A worrier. All of these factors play a part in my disorder, I learn afterward. The second day after taking my medication, my mind is on overdrive, and I am consumed with horrible thoughts.

It's three in the morning, and my husband is asleep in our bed. My mom is asleep in the room next to ours, and the baby is down the hall. My mind is full of terrifying thoughts that I might mindlessly black out and do something horrible. I don't know then that there are different types and levels to perinatal mood disorder. In a peak of panic, I make my mother get up and take me to her place in the next town over so that the baby will be safe. I lie awake waiting for daylight so that I can go to the doctor and beg for something to help me sleep.

The next few weeks are tumultuous as I slowly become re-balanced, rested, and calm. We find a wonderful support group right in my town called Adjustments After Birth. It is my safe haven. To meet other women just like me is a life preserver. Relief and gratitude flood my heart. I slowly work on healing myself and understanding what postpartum mood disorders are.

But I am very angry for a long time. *Why me? Why did something like this happen to me?* I am a strong, intellectual woman, and I wanted my baby. I have a desperate need to understand this volcanic explosion of panic and fear that hit me after I had my child. I begin to do research. I need to know the makeup of this illness. I get my answers, but there are no cut and dry reasons why I suffered from a perinatal mental illness. This is why I call it a spectrum disorder because the triggers are diverse and complicated. My history, my disposition, personality, my age, and the IVF were just a few of the factors. Each mother will have their own unique collection of triggers.

Understanding why this happened to me is important and necessary. This illness needs to be understood. Because I have such high empathy for mothers suffering the same trauma, I have become an advocate. I created my own website and Facebook page and took perinatal training. I have dreams of creating support centres and resources for moms and I hope one day these will be a reality. I am so grateful for my healing and I want mothers who are suffering to get the help they need, too.

Lisa Molinelli is mom to Aidan and lives in Caledon, Ontario She runs a Facebook Page for moms going through a perinatal mental illness @ittakesavillage4 and can be found on Instagram @lisa_molinelli

Motherhood, Anxiety, and Scary Thoughts

Karen Kleiman and Dr. Nichole Fairbrother

Mothering is hard. Anxiety can distort your thinking and convince you that you are out of control and you will always feel this way. You will not always feel like this.
- Karen Kleiman, *Good Moms Have Scary Thoughts*

Karen: Women have been telling me for over 35 years what they need and what they want to help them through some of the darkest days of their lives. Most of what I have learned has come from their hearts; much of what has been written in my books, has come directly from their voices. Perinatal women are uniquely attuned to what they feel and what they need. Their sensibilities are on hyper alert and most of the time, not always, but most of the time, they are very right about what they need and what they want, in order to heal. So, we should listen carefully.

But when it comes to scary thoughts, they are wrong. They are very wrong.

Because most perinatal women find it impossible to talk about the scary thoughts that they are having. The thoughts that drive a stake through their tender hearts and make them question whether or not they are fit to be a mother. But the paradox is, until they take the risk of sharing these thoughts, or images or impulses, the thoughts tend to get bigger, more powerful, and scarier for the women who experience them.

Nichole: While completing my PhD, I gave birth to my first child. I fell in love with my delightful son who is now a young adult, and the life-changing experience of pregnancy, birth, and parenting. At that time, I also experienced some out-of-the-blue thoughts that really startled me like, *I could throw my son out the window and go and make breakfast* and looking at my son's tiny fingers I thought, *they are so cute. I could cut them off with the garden clippers.*

Because I knew a lot about obsessive-compulsive disorder (OCD), I remember thinking, *Wow, that's so cool. I'm experiencing an unwanted, intrusive thought just like the kind that people with OCD experience and are so troubled by.* I knew that 85% of adults experience these kinds of thoughts, which, although unpleasant, are normal.

I then began to think about what it would be like if I didn't know anything about OCD, and I was a new mom alone at night with a crying infant. That would be so frightening. Once I began asking about this phenomenon, I learned that not only had very little research been conducted in this area, but some women who reported symptoms of postpartum OCD to their care providers had had their infant removed from their care from fear that they were at risk of abusing their child.

I knew right then that I needed to study this topic and make life better for pregnant and postpartum women suffering from these kinds of thoughts. For the past 15 years, my passion has been to improve the lives of pregnant and postpartum women who are suffering from anxiety, and in particular, OCD.

~

WE HAVE MADE MUCH PROGRESS in bringing public awareness and increased attention to the needs of new mothers. Despite this momentum in the right direction, our knowledge and understanding of postpartum harm thoughts lags behind.

The belief that all thoughts of infant-related harm represent a risk to infant safety is pervasive, and when women experience these kinds of thoughts, it is understandable that they are terrified that their infant could be removed from their care. Very little is known about these kinds of thoughts, and public education is lacking. As a result, most new mothers are not educated about them and are very isolated in their experience of them, often too fearful to disclose them to anyone.

What we now know, is that all new mothers experience some unwanted, intrusive thoughts of harm coming to their infant by accident (e.g., "What if my baby rolls off the bed?" "What if I trip while carrying my infant?"), and that 50% of new mothers experience unwanted, intrusive thoughts of harming their infant on purpose (e.g., "What if I shake my baby?" "What if I throw my baby out the window?"). Although thoughts of intentional harm are less common, not surprisingly, they are also more disturbing to the one experiencing them.

Postpartum women are frequently fearful of sharing these thoughts with others, partly because they fear that the fact that they are experiencing these kinds of thoughts might mean they are a bad or dangerous person, but also because they fear (with some justification) potential negative consequences such as monitoring for child abuse or removal of their infant from their care. They remain reluctant to tell anyone about the obsessive thoughts and the consuming guilt. Not even their partners. Instead, they pretend to be fine. They go to great lengths to look good and create the illusion that everything is in control. They often find it difficult to ask for help and spend a ton of energy making sure that everything appears perfect. If they are excessively concerned about their thoughts, they may also be at risk of developing mental health difficulties such as OCD or depression.

What are scary thoughts of infant-related harmand why do parents experience them?

All new mothers are anxious. All new fathers are anxious. Of course they are. There is so much to worry about at once. Anxiety is commonly understood to be a "normal" part of adjusting to this life-altering, exhilarating, exhausting, and overwhelming life transition. It is not surprising to most new parents that their lives will be uprooted for a while and in addition to the joy that comes with having a baby, there will be moments or days or weeks of chaos, strong conflicting emotions, and a flurry of confusing thoughts that make the most stable person wonder what the heck they got themselves into!

When stress is high, our survival response pumps adrenaline throughout our nervous system, which leads to an increase in heart rate, blood pressure and palpitations. This fight-or-flight response, an adaptive and instinctive response to perceived emotional or physical danger, is designed to keep us safe, aware, and prepared to take action. This primal reaction to excessive stress makes sense to most new parents who know, only too well, what it feels like to walk around in a chronic state of hyper-arousal. It feels important. It feels necessary. It feels exhausting.

It is also the case that the vast majority of adults (about 85%) report occasional thoughts (thoughts, images or impulses) that are intrusive and unwanted. We know that intrusive thoughts tend to occur more often when we are stressed and the content of these thoughts tends to revolve around the topics we are most concerned about. Given the ubiquity of information about potential risks to one's infant (e.g., crib safety, car seats, baby monitors, other accidents), it is not at all surprising that new mothers experience thoughts about harm coming to their infant, leading to all kinds of "what-ifs" and imagined horrific scenarios. Several scientists have hypothesized that the experience of harm thoughts related to one's infant may be adaptive in that they push parents to be more vigilant to sources of danger, and as a result, keep their infants safe. This is likely the case whether the thought is about accidental or intentional harm. Both "What if I trip and drop my baby?" and "What if I drop my baby on purpose?" are likely to lead to increased care. Even though the intention of doing harm will feel more stressful to the parent who experiences it, from an evolutionary perspective, it doesn't really matter if the thoughts are of accidental harm or intentional harm, as long as the result is increased attention to safety.

Understanding the nature of these thoughts

Unwanted, intrusive thoughts—typically about harm coming to one's infant are described aptly by Karen Kleiman (2020) as "scary thoughts." These kinds of thoughts, for some women, can be recurrent and associated with significant distress, leading understandably to feelings of guilt, shame, and self-loathing. The list of statements below is excerpted from Karen's book Dropping the Baby and Other Scary Thoughts (Kleiman et al, 2020) to help you get a snapshot of scary thoughts so you can put it in perspective and gain insight into how to manage your anxiety right now. These descriptions will help you understand what scary thoughts are and what they are not. Over the past 10 or more years various researchers (e.g., Drs. Nichole Fairbrother and Jonathon Abramowitz) have been studying postpartum UITs of infant-related harm (or scary thoughts) and here is what we now know:

- Scary thoughts are a normal (although really unpleasant) and common occurrence for almost all new moms and dads.
- Scary thoughts can come in the form of thoughts (what if I burn the baby in the bathtub?), images (an image of the baby falling

off the changing table), and impulses (the urge to scream at one's infant).

- Scary thoughts can be about accidental harm (something might happen to the baby) or intentional harm (thoughts or images of you throwing the baby against the wall)
- Scary thoughts of accidental harm are reported by 100% of new mothers.
- Scary thoughts of intentional harm are reported by 50% of new mothers.
- Scary thoughts are repetitive, unwanted, intrusive thoughts that can happen at any time.
- Scary thoughts don't need to be frightening—they are a normal part of early parenting.
- Scary thoughts only become a problem if new mothers who experience them interpret the thoughts to mean something terrible about themselves or their baby...For example: I am a crazy, bad or dangerous mom; or Something terrible is going to happen to my baby.
- Mothers make negative and frightening interpretations of their thoughts (probably because no one has told them that these kinds of thoughts are normal) are at increased risk for OCD and depression.
- If you have a history of OCD or tend to be a worrier or describe yourself as overly analytical or perfectionist, you may be at increased risk of developing OCD or depression in response to your scary thoughts.
- Scary thoughts typically focus on your baby, but can also center on thoughts about you, or your partner.
- Scary thoughts may be fleeting or they may race in your head throughout the day or keep you from falling asleep at night.
- Scary thoughts are not an indication of psychosis. They may make you feel like you are going crazy but you are not.
- Scary thoughts will make you feel like you're a bad parent. They will make you feel guilty and ashamed. Try not to beat yourself up about this. Remind yourself it is a common manifestation of anxiety.

Perhaps the single most powerful reminder, to help reduce your fear of scary thoughts is this:

There is NO relationship between a mother's scary thoughts and her taking any action in response to these thoughts.

In the one study (conducted by Nichole Fairbrother and her team), to have looked directly at this question, women who reported unwanted, intrusive thoughts of harming their baby on purpose were no more likely than women who only reported unwanted, intrusive thoughts of accidental harm coming to their infant to actually harm their infants (Fairbrother & Woody, 2008).

It is easy to see how overwhelming a new parent might feel when they unexpectedly experience such abhorrent notions, but that's exactly why it's important that you are informed. Your fear does not mean anything terrible is happening. It just feels that way. And it feels that way to most new parents at some point in time or another. Scary thoughts are so common in new parents that when we provide professional training, we tell healthcare providers to expect these high levels of distress in new parents. Medical providers should look for it, screen for it, and be prepared with a list of local resources to support every new parent. Research by Jon Abramowitz (Abramowitz, 2006) found that 91% of all new moms (not just those diagnosed with postpartum depression or anxiety) and 88% of all new dads experienced negative intrusive thoughts about harm coming to their babies. Nichole Fairbrother's team has found that 100% of new mothers report thoughts of accidental harm related to the newborn, and 50% report thoughts of intentional harm (Fairbrother & Woody, 2008). That means almost every single new parent experiences these kinds of thoughts! That is how universal this phenomenon is. Still, if you are someone who is not able to brush off these scary thoughts or if they are so pervasive or so disturbing that you are not reassured by this information and feel something is terribly wrong, please let your healthcare provider know how you feel. It is worth noting that a majority of women discover that when they talk about what they are feeling and thinking in a safe environment with someone who understands that this is a common occurrence, they feel better. Their anxiety decreases.

Are postpartum scary thoughts related to a mothers' mental health?

When most people learn that a mother is experiencing unwanted, intrusive thoughts of harm related to her infant, their first concern is for the infant and they worry the mother may be at risk of harming her infant. While it is true that in very rare cases some women may be at risk of harming their infants (e.g., if they are experiencing postpartum psychosis), what we now know is that there is no evidence that the experience of unwanted, intrusive thoughts, images and impulses of harming one's infant on purpose is a risk factor for child abuse.

However, postpartum harm thoughts may be a risk factor for the development or exacerbation of obsessive-compulsive disorder. OCD is an anxiety-related disorder characterized by two types of symptoms: (a) obsessions (recurrent, unwanted and distressing thoughts, images, or impulses), and (b) compulsions (repetitive mental or physical behaviors that the person engages in, in order to feel less upset about the obsessions). The content of obsessions typically involves thoughts that are about contamination, violence, sex, religion, and/or being responsible for harm to others (e.g., one's baby). The compulsive behaviors associated with the obsessions typically involve checking (e.g., checking on one's baby), reassurance seeking (looking things up on the internet), washing and cleaning rituals (excessive washing of the baby, or possessions related to the baby), and repetitive mental acts (e.g., visualizing one's baby breathing and well). It is also common for people suffering from OCD to avoid situations related to the content of their obsessions.

OCD sufferers, due to the fact that their obsessions are often socially unacceptable in nature, are frequently motivated to conceal their obsessions from others, including health-care providers. This is especially true for new mothers who are experiencing obsessions related to their infant. Current theories of how OCD develops hypothesize that unwanted, intrusive thoughts are a common and normal human experience. However, if the person experiencing these thoughts interprets the fact that they are experiencing them, and/or the content of the thoughts to mean something bad about themselves (e.g., "The fact that I am having these thoughts means that I am a bad, dangerous or crazy mother.") or their future (e.g., "These thoughts mean that my baby may be harmed.") they may be at risk of developing OCD. Women who are vulnerable to making these kinds of appraisals are more likely to experience OCD during pregnancy and postpartum.

There is now very strong evidence that the perinatal period, in particular, the postpartum period, is a time of high risk for the development or worsening of OCD. This is particularly true for first time parents. This is likely due to the fact that the perinatal period is characterized by a dramatic increase in (a) feelings of responsibility (i.e., "I am fully responsible for my infant.") and (b) threat ("What if something happens to my baby?"). These factors make it more likely that new parents will misinterpret normally occurring intrusive "scary" thoughts to mean something threatening.

What you can do to help yourself feel better?

If you are worried about the thoughts you are having, that's a good sign. Of course you're worried. It's excruciatingly painful to feel so attached and loving toward your baby and have such scary thoughts at the same time. Having these thoughts make most moms feel guilty, ashamed and scared of what it means. You are probably thinking something like: A good mother wouldn't think such awful things. But good mothers do think bad thoughts. In fact, when Karen wrote Good Moms Have Scary Thoughts (Kleiman, 2019), the title was initially rejected by the publisher because it sounded harsh and negative. Scary, almost. They were later convinced that this is precisely the point; that the objective was to state outright, with transparency, that this phenomenon is real, it is common, and we need to address it without sugarcoating it so women can be informed.

For women who interpret these thoughts to mean something frightening for themselves or their infants, in particular women who struggle with symptoms of depression and anxiety, scary thoughts become exaggerated, persistent, and hard to shake. If these thoughts do not feel consistent with who you are, if they seem totally out of character for you, or if you know they are irrational and make no sense, it shows that the thoughts are a normal postpartum experience, and not psychosis. Remember that these thoughts are not about who you are. They are a normal and unpleasant postpartum experience. Again, if your distress is high, it is a good idea to seek support and professional resources to help reframe your response to them. In the meantime, there are things you can do to minimize your distress.

Let's start with what will NOT help you feel better

As first described in Dropping the Baby and Other Scary Thoughts (Kleiman et al, 2020), the following eight principles should underscore the way you think and respond to any scary thoughts you are having:

- Denying the feelings and thoughts will not make them go away.
- Panicking will make it worse.
- Resistance creates persistence.
- Distraction will help for a while.
- Enhancing awareness might feel counterintuitive, but it is meaningful.
- Acceptance is hard but essential.
- Letting others know can ease the burden.

Moreover, there is evidence that the following four responses, while common, are actually maladaptive and can intensity an already anxious reaction:

1. **Denial:** Pretending or behaving as if the thoughts are not there will unexpectedly make them more powerful.
2. **Thought suppression:** A common reaction to such disturbing thoughts is to wish them away. Actually, trying to control the thoughts by hiding them or suppressing them can end up backfiring.
3. **Safety-seeking behaviors:** The problem with seeking reassurance is that it only helps for a brief period. The more you engage in this behavior to seek reassurance and certainty the more anxious it makes you feel. Learning to tolerate uncertainty is extremely difficult and extremely important. Everyone can relate to the temptation to google something only to find yourself feeling

worse after reading some catastrophic possibility that is unrelated to what you were looking up in the first place! Stay off the Internet.

4. **Panic:** High anxiety can cause scary thoughts to emerge and scary thoughts can cause you to panic. Rather than think, "Well, that was a weird thought" and dismiss it as annoying, panic forces you to fixate on the thought, or on how bad it feels, or on how crazy it makes you think you are. Obsessing on the scary thought is exhausting and unproductive.

While the above behaviors and responses to anxiety might provide some initial decrease in distress, they also bring more attention to the intrusive thoughts which serves to empower and negatively reinforce them.

How you think can get in the way

While it's understandable that you would be unsettled by your negative thoughts, learning how to respond to them in more productive ways is likely to minimize their impact and reduce your anxiety.

1. **Normalize:** Perhaps the single most important thing you can do with your scary thoughts is to accept that they are common and normal (yes, they feel awful) and that they don't mean anything about you as a mother.
2. **False alarm:** When we experience a scary thought, at first, our alarm bells go off and we feel afraid. The most important thing you can do is to remember that this is a FALSE ALARM! Your unwanted, intrusive thoughts of harm related to your baby, are NOT DANGEROUS.
3. **Accept:** When your thoughts occur, recognize that they are unpleasant, acknowledge that they don't tell you anything negative about yourself as a parent (they do tell you that your baby's safety is really important to you) and DON'T PUSH THEM AWAY—Notice them and just let them be. Pushing them away can increase how often you have them and this can make you very anxious.

4. **Do nothing:** This sounds counter-intuitive, but one of the worst things you can do is behave as if the thoughts are meaningful. So, DO NOT respond to your thoughts with checking or washing or other actions to make sure the thought isn't a warning about danger! Often, when new mothers have a thought about danger related to their baby, they want to do lots and lots of checking! It's okay to check on your baby once, but repeated checking can actually increase your anxiety.
5. **OCD thinking:** Interventions and strategies for relief which we suggest for scary thoughts, apply to everyone, but if you have OCD it may be more challenging for you to do by yourself and it can also be a little more complicated. Cognitive behavioral therapy (CBT) is the most scientifically supported form of therapy for OCD. Seek the help of a cognitive behavioral therapist. Even better if you can work with a CBT therapist with experience in treating perinatal OCD.

Strategies for relief

1. **Distraction strategies:** Distraction really does help. When your brain is busy focusing on something else, perhaps something particularly soothing or painstakingly tedious, it interrupts your negative ruminations. Distracting examples are endless. Find what works best for you. For example: Reading, dancing, listening to music, organizing, playing games, doing puzzles, exercising, call a friend, to name only a few.
2. **Self-regulation strategies:** Mindfulness, relaxation, breathing: As described in Dropping the Baby and Other Scary Thoughts (Kleiman et al, 2020), breathing, relaxation and mindfulness practice can help you feel more in control and teach you skills that will improve your body's reactions to stress. One of the reasons anxiety is so uncomfortable is because it upsets the entire body: Your heart starts racing, your breathing is shallow, and your body feels tense and on high alert. Anxiety can deplete your energy and make you feel tired, irritable and unable to concentrate. This is why the majority of

anti-anxiety strategies focus on techniques to help your body relax. Relaxation exercises can weaken the stress response and neutralize physical tension. In a relaxed state, the nervous system unwinds which leads to a slower heart rate, more controlled breathing, and a stabilization of blood pressure. You can see how all of these self-regulating strategies, such as mindfulness, relaxation and breathing exercises, overlap and work together to calm the body and quiet the restless mind. **Mindfulness** refers to the mental practice of becoming more aware of your present state and learning how to accept your thoughts and emotions, without reacting to them. This involves learning how to pay attention differently and with intention and is most successful after refinement through regular practice. **Relaxation** refers to a more physical practice, in response to bodily functions and sensations with an attempt to regulate or modify some of our natural states that might be dysregulated by acute or chronic anxiety. **Deep Breathing,** an essential component of both mindfulness and relaxation, refers to the slow, abdominal intake and exhaling breath through the nose. Deep breathing has been shown to increase oxygen to the brain, slow the heartbeat and lower and stabilize blood pressure.

3. **Self-Care Strategies:**

   Journaling: Sometimes, the best thing you can do for yourself when anxiety is high is to identify it and put words to it. Journaling has been shown to help this process by allowing you to bring it out from under the shadow of shame and into your awareness in a way that is purposeful and focused on your mental, emotional, and physical well-being.

   S.E.L.F.: At The Postpartum Stress Center, we use the acronym S.E.L.F. to remind moms to pay attention to what their bodies need. Sleep: We know that sleep is at a premium right now, but rearranging things to help accommodate your need for sleep should be a priority when possible.

   Exercise: While this isn't new information, a recent study does shed new light on the relationship between movement and mood.

While it was still recommended that you do at least 15 minutes of intense exercise, such as running, or an hour of lower-intensity exercise, such as walking or housework, the authors point out that any intentional moving of the body, such as stair-climbing, or cleaning, can help lift the mood (Choi, 2019). The conclusion was: People who move more had a lower risk for depression.

Laugh: Studies have shown that laughter can enhance the immune system and activate the release of endorphins, which can improve mood. It can also ease tension in the body.

Food: Modifying your diet can help reduce anxiety symptoms. Don't forget to stay hydrated and avoid alcohol and caffeine. Both have the potential to exacerbate anxiety and interfere with sleep.

Support Groups: The success of support groups, like anything else, is dependent on many variables, most of which, are out of your control. Factors include, who is the facilitator? What is their training? Who is sponsoring the group? Who are the group members? To what degree are they struggling? To what degree do their personalities and preferences drive the dynamics of the group? Ultimately, it depends how the group experience feels to you. Generally speaking, support groups have proven to be a reliable option for mild-to-moderate anxiety and depressive symptoms. They can be enormously comforting and provide the opportunity for much needed interactions and validation. They can also serve to reduce the stigma and help defuse some of the myths about scary thoughts, particularly when psychoeducation is presented.

With any of these self-help strategies, keep in mind how you are feeling and try your best to monitor how you respond to these interventions. If your symptoms of anxiety cause interference in your life, a professional support might be a better choice for symptom relief. As mentioned throughout this chapter, anxiety feeds off of your reaction and interpretation of it. Your fear and resistance will magnify the distress. Your acceptance of the distress will help you gain some semblance of control, which, ultimately, feels better..

Final Thoughts on Regaining a Sense of Control

- **The Way Back to Yourself:** You will not always feel this way. You have more power over the way you feel than you might believe. Remember, as Karen always reminds moms: these scary thoughts are symptoms, they are not who you are. As your anxiety is managed, either by you or by professional treatment, these thoughts will subside and their power over you will decrease. The key is to accept that they are there for now, and try hard to move forward despite them.
- **Do not do this alone:** Find a safe person you can trust and let them know how you feel. Share some reliable resources with them so they are adequately informed and can continue to provide the support you need. Let your healthcare provider know how you feel. Download helpful information from reputable websites or carry a copy of Good Moms Have Scary Thoughts with you! Make sure the professionals who are treating you have access to accurate information. There is no reason why you cannot help them help you! If your distress remains high and you feel that your symptoms interfere with your day, finding a therapist who specializes in the treatment of prenatal and postpartum (perinatal) mood and anxiety disorders (PMADs) can help enormously.
- **Believe in your ability to heal:** When you're overwhelmed, consumed by worry, and sleep-deprived, believing in yourself can feel like an impossibility. Nonetheless, it's important to dig deep and find moments of self-compassion to help buoy you as you navigate this challenging time in your life. While your instinct to judge yourself harshly may be your automatic response, it will not help you feel better. Instead, find ways to be gentler with yourself and believe that you can learn the skills to help yourself through this with self-compassion and acceptance. You will feel better again.

Karen Kleiman is a well-known international maternal mental health expert, with over 35 years of experience. As an advocate and author of several groundbreaking books on postpartum depression and anxiety, her pioneering work continues to inspire moms, perinatal therapists, and the maternal mental health community across the globe. In 1988, Karen founded The Postpartum Stress Center, a premier treatment and training facility for prenatal and postpartum depression/anxiety disorders. Find the Postpartum Stress Center on Facebook and Twitter @ ppstresscenter and on Instagram @postpartumstress which includes the #speakthesecret campaign to bust the stigma of perinatal intrusive thoughts.

Dr. Nichole Fairbrother is director of the Perinatal Anxiety Research Lab at the University of British Columbia. Dr. Fairbrother is a Clinical Associate Professor in the University of British Columbia's Department of Psychiatry, and a member of the Women's Health Research Institute at B.C. Women's Hospital. Dr. Fairbrother's research is in the area of reproductive mental health with a focus on new mothers' thoughts of infant-related harm and OCD. More information about Dr. Fairbrother's work can be found on her website at www.parlab.ubc.ca

WHITE-KNUCKLING IT

Heather Marcoux

I SLID DOWN THE BATHROOM wall, my baby strapped to my chest and hung up the phone. It had taken me weeks to gather up my courage and call the mental health department, but I was transferred from a human to a recorded voice reading out addresses. I couldn't keep going. I put the phone down and cried, again.

Coming to terms with how motherhood impacted my mental health (and the other way around) was a long process made harder, in my opinion, by a health care system that wasn't interested in meeting my needs.

When I was pregnant, I would lay in bed long past my alarm, until the sun shone through the window, and text my boss, *I can't make it in today—too sick.* I'm sure he assumed I was talking about the morning sickness that had plagued me for months, but that wasn't the kind of sickness I had.

I was physically fine and emotionally spent. I just wanted to stay in my blankets and imagine what a great life this baby would have without me. Imagine the woman my husband could find after my inevitable death.

I did reach out for help when I was pregnant. I told my doctor, "I cry every day. I can't stop." She laughed and said, "That's just part of being pregnant."

I tried to track down the email of the nurse at the primary care network had given me—the one who told me to reach out if I ever needed someone—but no one answering the phone knew who I was talking about and I'd lost her card.

Thankfully, in the third trimester, my mood improved drastically. I was able to get up and move and nest and was so looking forward to meeting my baby. And when I did, it was incredible.

When the health nurse came to check on my family two days after we came home from the hospital, she remarked on how great I looked, that most moms weren't able to get dressed and do their hair this early. I even had makeup on.

I rode that new-mom high for months. I was great at this. I was back to walking my dogs just days after giving birth. I was a superhero. And so I passed the mental health assessment at my child's first health unit appointment. I was fine.

But then the darkness came back. I was tired, so incredibly tired, and I began to think sad thoughts. Complex thoughts. Thoughts like I need to find new homes for my dogs because if my husband's a widower and a single dad, he won't be able to handle them. Maybe he can keep the cat.

The day before my baby's second health unit appointment I got so excited. *They're gonna do the mental health screen again*, I thought. *She'll see I need help.* But when we got to the appointment they didn't do the screening. I'd passed the last time, so I guess that counted forever. Except everything had changed for me. And no one knew.

I went on like this for a long time, too long.

Finally, I went to the walk-in clinic and asked the doctor for help. They suggested I try a book on Amazon before antidepressants. I ordered the book. It had the word happy in the title but it didn't make me happier (perhaps because I put it in the breadbox instead of reading it).

I went back to the clinic and demanded antidepressants. I found a therapist through my husband's employee assistance plan. I got better, but this doesn't feel like a story about a mother finding support when she needed it. It feels like the story of a woman who white-knuckled her way into survival.

When my son was two, I got a job as the news editor for a popular mom brand, and I learned a lot about perinatal mental health. I learned about how depression is the most common complication of pregnancy, and about how one in five pregnant people experience depression. I learned about how prenatal depression is linked to developmental issues in children, and when my child experienced developmental issues, I blamed myself.

The mom guilt was overwhelming when my child was diagnosed with autism at age three, and for the second time in my motherhood, I sought therapy. This time I found a therapist who specialized in moms. For three sessions, I told her about my guilt and how I refused to let debunked junk science make me feel more guilt.

She told me that she didn't vaccinate her own children because she was afraid of what happened to mine. She told me my depression very well may have impacted my child's brain. It didn't feel particularly helpful.

I still went back to that therapist for several more sessions, even though my husband begged me not to because, sadly, she was the best mental health support I had found in three years. Eventually, I quit seeing her, because I couldn't forgive myself while sitting across from someone I perceived to be sitting in judgment of my depression and my choice to vaccinate my baby.

This sucked. Becoming a mom in a society that wouldn't give me a lifeline sucked. I don't know how to explain it any differently. Today, I have a new therapist and an (old, male) psychiatrist who doesn't understand the problems of modern motherhood at all but agrees to up the antidepressant dose whenever I ask.

I am disappointed in our society. I am not disappointed in myself. This—none of it, not the depression, not my baby's diagnosis, not the system failures—is my fault. But I am speaking out now for all the moms who don't know that it is not their fault. They're being told every day that they are failing when in reality, the system is failing us.

My baby is now five. We're no longer on the bathroom floor. And I don't want to see anyone else down there.

Heather Marcoux is a mom to one little boy and lives in Red Deer, Alberta. An award-winning journalist, Heather has worked for Canada's biggest broadcasters and in American print and digital media. You can find her on Twitter @heathermarcoux

BEHIND THE SCENES

Leigh Mitchell

I'M GRATEFUL TO BE A mother. I have two amazing boys. However, my journey into motherhood was not as smooth as I expected.

I always knew that having children could be life-changing, but I didn't anticipate what would happen to me before, during, and after my first pregnancy. My diagnosis of postpartum depression came as the biggest shock of new motherhood. What followed was a long journey to recovery, and a critical part of that would be creating an active lifestyle for my baby and me.

My journey began before I even had my son. It started with severe anxiety around doctors' appointments and obsessions over baby gates. One of my friends who was already a mom laughed at me, saying I wouldn't need a baby gate until six months after I gave birth, but I continued with my obsessive thinking patterns.

Then came a rough delivery. My son was delivered by emergency C-section, after which I mourned not having a *natural birth* I never got to experience. When it came time to leave the hospital, I was so afraid that I asked not to be discharged. I was unprepared for the post-surgery pain I felt and was freaking out about not having mastered breastfeeding yet.

Behind the scenes, my husband reassured the nurses that I was okay and that we would all feel better once we were settled at home. I arrived home to find my mother-in-law waiting in the driveway with food, balloons, and well wishes.

That night, I had my first panic attack. I thought I was having a heart attack. The next day, a public health nurse visited our home. She reassured me that I didn't have a heart problem, and informed me that it was likely a panic attack.

The nurse visit was part of a City of Toronto program that provided support to new moms. Sadly, it didn't include any pamphlets or information on postpartum depression. It would be a long time before I figured out that I had postpartum depression—and only because my cousin made me see my family doctor.

By my six-week postpartum checkup, I knew something was wrong. I was having difficulty sleeping when my baby son slept, and I felt like I was slowly going insane. Panic attacks became more frequent. I confided in my obstetrician, but unfortunately, and somewhat shockingly, she was not trained to recognize or support perinatal mental illness. Now I didn't know where to turn.

I confided in my mom and my husband, but I felt like they didn't understand what I was experiencing and that they were making light of it. Everyone around me seemed to be in denial. They figured that being a new parent was tough for anyone, so feeling down was just normal and not necessarily a sign of depression. But my cousin, also a new mom, knew me well, and she could see that something was wrong.

With my cousin's encouragement, I went to see my family doctor, and I was finally diagnosed with postpartum depression. I started taking medication, and began to slowly feel like my old self again. Even on medication, I was able to continue to breastfeed safely. I became able to sleep when my baby was sleeping and I felt a lot better. Still, I discovered that being a new mom was very isolating, and that made recovery hard.

I remember calling my husband the day he returned to work, telling him I was lonely. I joked that I wanted him to stay at home and let me go back to work.

I soon discovered that the key to not feeling isolated was actually pretty simple: I needed to get out and meet other new parents. I started going to the Ontario Early Years Centres with my son and participated in baby and me exercise classes. I also joined a support group for postpartum depression. Through all of these activities, I made new friends who joined me for walks and visits to storytime at the library and bookstore.

It made a huge difference. The health benefits of our shared exercise proved to be great for my son and me. It reduced my anxiety, and I found that he was less fussy and slept better.

In the end, I conquered my postpartum depression and became a confident and happy mother. However, it was a long and difficult journey and one that could have been easier if more support had been available to me from the beginning. I'm stronger for this experience. I don't regret having lived with postpartum depression—it helped me to find my voice, fine-tune my priorities, and ultimately increased the bonds I have with my family.

Leigh Mitchell is a mom of two and lives in Toronto, Ontario. Leigh is the founder of Women in Biz Network and is passionate about mental health advocacy. Connect with Leigh on all your favourite social media platforms @womenbiznetwork

MAMAHOOD: BURSTING INTO LIGHT

Nicolle Nattrass

HERE HE IS, IN HIS crib, lying so beautiful, so trusting with the face of an angel. I am so scared something's going to happen to him.

I am scared at night. My thoughts are so loud.

You can't do this right. He'd be better off without you.

My mind starts moving backwards in time, fast. It won't stop. I go back in time to every mistake.

Every relationship break-up. Every friend that I had a falling out with. Every time I did anything wrong.

I'm back in grade five. At a sleepover. It's the middle of the night and my sleeping bag is rolled back. I look up and someone is standing over me. Someone starts touching me. I want to say stop. But I don't.

I never tell anyone.

I look down at my beautiful baby, so pure, so perfect.

Oh god. I'm failing. I'm failing at this. I can't fail at this.

I do what I always do to get through. What any self-respecting, god-fearing person would do.

I pull out my old David Bowie records.

But seriously, I'm caught in this loop—angry, scared, can't sleep, angry, scared, can't sleep. I don't feel like myself. I don't talk to my partner anymore. Everything makes me irritated and angry.

I slam doors. I yell and then look down and see his face.

This tiny face.

I can't do this anymore.

I call the child resource centre. I need help. They arrange for a home visit.

A couple days later, the doorbell rings.

"I'll be right there!" I yell out.

I open the door and Barbara, the woman from the child resource centre is there. Before she can say anything, I blurt out: "Hi, sorry, the power just went out and I'm in the middle of cooking pancakes. My baby is screaming for his fancy pancakes!"

"Alright, then would you like to reschedule? I can come back at another time?" Barbara asks.

I really want to cancel but something inside me says I'd better not.

"No, of course not. Come on in!" I say.

She sits on the couch. I sit on the floor in front of her. Never in my life has my house been so disorganized, my hair so ratty, and my outfit so freaking uncoordinated.

"How are you doing?" Barbara asks.

"I'm great! You?" I respond.

Was I just yelling? Yes I was. *Keep your voice down,* I tell myself, *or you'll scare the nice lady away.* She seems like a nice little grandma. Then I look at her again and she looks like the psychic lady from the movie *Poltergeist. Go into the light, Carol Ann. Go into the light.* Oh god, I am really losing it!

"And who is this, might I ask?" asks Barbara.

"Mario. His name is Mario," I say.

"Beautiful name," says Barbara.

She plays with him for a little while then asks if it's alright if she comes back and sees him again.

"Sure, I guess," I say.

The following week, she's back, playing on the floor with him again.

"He is doing really well. I'm not seeing signs of any hyper activity or any other markers we need to be concerned about. His vocabulary is very advanced, over 400 words. He loves to talk," Barbara says.

"How are you feeling, Nicolle?"

"Me? Oh I'm fine," I respond back.

"Did you get a call from the public health nurse?"

"No. Yes, yes, I do remember talking to someone," I say.

"Did she go over the checklist with you for postpartum depression?" Barbara inquires.

"Yes. I scored within the normal range. I'm pretty strong. I don't think I can get it." I inform Barbara.

"How would you describe Mario's sleeping patterns?" asks Barbara.

"He has slept through the night, I don't know, about six times," I say.

"In two years? You have to get your rest. Prolonged sleep deprivation is very serious. It's very detrimental to your health, mentally and physically. I want to help. Maybe we can develop a new routine together so he can sleep for longer periods."

"Okay, yes, but I'm not leaving him to cry it out," I say to Barbara.

"That's fine. I can give you some other tools. Do you mind me asking you about the birth?"

I tell her about my traumatic labour experience.

"Have you heard of post-traumatic stress disorder?" asks Barbara.

"PTSD? Yes I've heard of it," I reply.

"It can happen to women who have had difficult births, too. You may be experiencing some of the symptoms. I'll bring you some literature to read."

For the first time, I start to read about the baby blues, postpartum depression, and postpartum-traumatic stress disorder. I find I can relate to a combination of them all. Maybe that's why I'm so scared at night and these memories are coming back.

Mario likes Barbara. I like her too. She is like a beacon. She listens to both Mario and me. No judgments. No manuals. No magic formulas.

I am able to get help for PTSD and things start looking up. Mario's sleep improves, and I begin feeling more and more like myself again.

One day, we decide to go on a family trip. It's my birthday and we go to the Vancouver Aquarium. I'm half listening because I'm thinking we need to do a diaper change soon but I can hear the marine assistant describing the dolphins, who are rescues. One has scars, the other's fin was cut off by a boat rudder.

The dolphins burst out of the water together, and I can't take my eyes off them. I can see their scars glistening in the sun. It's like I'm coming out of the water, too, and out of the dark and seeing everything around me for the first time. I look over at my boy, his beautiful face, and he says, "Mama, why are you crying?"

"Because I am happy Mario! You make me so happy!"

I smile more. I play more. I feel like maybe I'm not failing. I notice things again. Mario and I go for walks together and I point out the birds and the blackberries. I can laugh again. I start to talk to my partner more. We aren't galaxies apart. I reach out to him in the chaos in between the dirty dishes and the avocado bits. "Hey, I think you are kinda cute. Have we met before?"

I'm me again. Sort of fragile. Sort of different—but still me. I am bursting into light.

Nicolle Nattrass is a Jessie Award nominated actress (CAEA/ACTRA), playwright (PGC), counsellor CAC II and instructor for Creative Journaling for Self-Care. Nicolle began keeping a journal of her experience as a new mother and those notes became an autobiographical 90-minute one-woman play that she performed in theatres since 2016. Her play, *Mamahood: Bursting into Light* is a witty and profoundly moving ode to motherhood. Connect with Nicolle on Instagram @nicollenattrass2019 or through her website at www.nicollenattrass.com

WORTHY OF LOVE

Stephanie George

I LOVE BEING A MOM. Being a mom to my two kids brings me purpose, happiness, and makes me feel like I am doing something important. Being a mom is the highlight of my life.

I try so hard to be the best mom, the best wife, and the best daughter. I do what is expected of me, no matter the time of day or night. I keep the peace. I think that's what I have to do.

My husband was finishing college and working part time while I was pregnant with baby number three. One day, while watching something on TV with my boys, I had a vision of throwing the youngest one, then two years old, through the window. I was terrified. Seeing that vision, and the many times I saw it later, scared the life out of me.

I was also cranky and not sleeping well. No one suggested that I could be anxious or depressed.

I fought my husband on using a midwife for my third pregnancy. It was one of the few times I put my foot down. He didn't trust their care so decided having a midwife birth—in hospital—was the only way he'd let it happen.

Luke's birth was beautiful. I was happy and doing well. Even my husband was in a kind of honeymoon state for a week after the experience. I hoped, deep down in a place I couldn't give voice to, that the positive changes in myself and in my mental health would be permanent.

They weren't.

At my six-week postpartum follow-up appointment, I told my midwife I'd been having trouble breathing and that I wasn't sure what was happening to me. I was diagnosed with asthma as a teen, so I thought perhaps it was acting up again.

My midwife opened up a small, purple book, and asked me to read a particular page while she left the office for a few minutes.

What I read changed my life.

It was about anxiety attacks. I could have written the signs and symptoms on my own. This was what I was experiencing back in my teen years, but, since the tests were indeterminate, it was chalked up to asthma. I always wondered why the puffers made my heart race more than help me breathe.

Anxiety.

I trusted her and told her about those thoughts I had of throwing my beautiful boy through our window. Was I going to be locked up for that? Was she going to call Child Protective Services? Was I going to lose my children? I was terrified. But...I trusted her.

"How do you feel when you see that?" she asked me.

"I hate it! It terrifies me! I feel like the world's worst mother," I replied, with tears streaming down my cheeks.

"I'm glad you feel horrible. That means it will never happen," she said.

She opened the book to a page about intrusive thoughts, and I read and I read and I read.

The little purple book helped me to see that I had been battling depression and anxiety since the middle of my pregnancy.

Shortly thereafter, we moved our family across the country to mountainous Telkwa, BC because my husband had gotten a job there. There seemed to be far less sunshine, and we knew no one.

I was still newly treating my postpartum anxiety and depression. The negative thoughts hadn't subsided yet. I had to stop myself from looking down the mountains because I had visions of me in the car, rolling down the cliffs. Strangely, these thoughts brought me peace.

I buried everything inside and didn't tell anyone because there were things to get done. The house had to be unpacked, the children had to be tended to, and we needed clean clothes and food to eat. I tried but my husband kept telling me how much of a failure I was. And I believed him.

One Saturday, after being in our new home for two months or so, I couldn't get off of the couch. The baby wanted to nurse and cried because I couldn't give him what he wanted. The older kids wanted to play with their mom, too. It was a terrible Saturday. My husband was working.

When he came home, he saw my distress. He suggested that I go for a ride to relax. Grateful for the time away, I put my coat and boots on and started to leave when he stopped me.

"Aren't you going to bring the baby?" he asked.

I wasn't going to because I was hoping for some alone time, but I dutifully packed up Luke and started the drive out to Smithers, a town roughly ten minutes away. I was crying but the baby was quiet.

Just outside of Telkwa limits, I started to wonder about which route to take.

Right or left?

If I drove into Smithers and turned right, I could take the car, me, and the baby down the cliff.

If I drove toward Smithers but turned left, I could try to find this old shack I saw when I was there ten years earlier. I just wanted to see if it had fallen flat by then or not. I believe the Creator put me on a high school trip I should never have been on for me to see that shack...so it would save my life a decade later.

Right or left?

It felt like the biggest decision and the longest moment of my life.

I believed that if I turned right, I would be making the best choice for everyone. My husband could find a new woman who brought him happiness, who could keep a cleaner house, and who could be a better mom. The only thing at that moment I believed I was good at was breast-feeding.

Right or left?

I turned left.

I stopped the car and sobbed. I hugged baby Luke like I had never hugged him before and nursed him until he fell asleep.

I put myself back together, drove home, thanked my husband for allowing me that time, and went back to living, knowing I wasn't doing any more than surviving.

I told my husband three weeks later about what happened that day on the road to Smithers. He was shocked, angry, and expressed concern. He forced me to go to the doctor, and I started taking medication to help with my anxiety attacks.

I wanted someone to talk to but couldn't find anyone, so I pushed the pregnancy centre to start up a postpartum depression support group. They did, but unfortunately, the woman in charge of the group hadn't healed from her own postpartum depression. We supported her more than ourselves.

My husband was supportive, to a point. He would walk in the door and say, "Oh, good, you're still alive. You have no idea how hard it is for me to worry about if you're going to be alive when I come home or not."

A year or so later, when I had started to feel better, I was asked to take part in a postpartum depression support person training. The trainers were from the organization that wrote the little purple book, the Pacific Postpartum Support Society. I jumped at the chance to give back and help other women going through the same struggles I did.

My story is not unique. Many Indigenous women suffer from postpartum mood and anxiety disorders. But in our communities, there is a greater stigma towards mental illness. I was once told by a Grandmother in the middle of my perinatal presentation that she didn't have time to be depressed back in her day.

Indigenous mothers are 20% more likely to suffer from prenatal and postpartum depression than white, Caucasian mothers in Canada. (https://pubmed.ncbi.nlm.nih.gov/30068224/) The findings parallel the Government of Canada's 2008 Maternity Experiences Survey that found Indigenous women have a higher prevalence of postpartum depression than non-Indigenous women. (https://www.canada.ca/en/public-health/services/reports-publications/health-promotion-chronic-disease-prevention-canada-research-policy-practice/vol-38-no-7-8-2018/mental-health-indeators-pregnant-aboriginal-women-maternity-experiences-survey.html)

Pregnant Indigenous women and service providers were interviewed for a 2015 Voices and PHACES study in Calgary, Alberta. The study found chronic life stress and trauma to be key causes of prenatal depression in Indigenous women. Almost all of the pregnant Indigenous women interviewed for the study reported being deeply and negatively impacted by having someone in their life—a parent, an aunt or uncle, a grandparent, an older sibling—who survived the Residential School system. (https://policywise.com/wp-content/uploads/resources/2016/07/2212015-11NOV-10_Final_Report_1_3_25_11SM-Thurston.pdf)

My mom was a product of the foster care system. Her father went to a Residential School outside of Brantford, Ontario. Residential Schools were government-supported religious schools developed to assimilate Indigenous children into Euro-Canadian culture. She was kind of like a "Sixties Scoop" child, which refers to an awful time during the 1960s when the government scooped Indigenous children from their homes to be adopted by mostly non-Indigenous, middle-class families in Canada and the U.S.

Among the recommendations stemming from the report include the creation of Indigenous-specific prenatal and parenting programs to address the intergenerational effects of Residential School trauma.

We have been a people surviving through dysfunction. There are families who have depression but will not name it. We feel silenced. We feel we don't have worth. We look for ways to heal but sometimes, it feels easier to stay in a situation where, even though we know it is unhealthy, we stay so we won't be alone.

We are told family is everything. Some of us are told that the man makes the rules. We chose (even if it wasn't a choice) to have our baby with him so we need to make it work. As the woman, it is our responsibility to make him happy. That dysfunction has been passed down from generation to generation.

I promised myself when I became an Indigenous midwife that I would always help Indigenous women to feel they are not alone. I help them to see and believe they are worthy of happiness. By them being happy, they will become moms who are more present for their children. They can start to see and feel their worth.

The women I work with are relieved when someone believes them, that they are able to speak with someone like who suffered from prenatal and postpartum depression and anxiety. They feel validated, accepted, and loved. Some of my clients changed their own trajectories and left their partners to start again in peace, in love, and in belief in themselves.

These women believe in themselves. They want a better future for their children. They want their children to be raised by a healthy mom.

Indigenous women are at the bottom of all social determinants of health in Canada. Statistics prove it study after study (and we are tired of being studied).

Studies about Indigenous issues tend to focus on how hard done we are, how we are impoverished and under employed, how sad we are to be in the scheme of things. Studies show how bad things are for us.

We need to change that.

We need studies to show our resiliency in the face of racist words, racist actions, systemic oppressions, patriarchal laws that inhabit our communities as we are all finding our strength as Indigenous communities as a whole.

When women feel supported by their families and their communities, we can heal. When we feel our own strength, we are unstoppable.

We need to hear stories of women who overcame their perinatal mental illness. We need to celebrate them. We need to see this in studies and in our communities.

We, as Indigenous women, are afraid to speak. Society, while making advances, still doesn't like hearing from us. Racism is rampant. We don't feel like we matter because we are told that. That also drives perinatal mental illness in our communities.

I am healing because people helped me to see my strength. They helped me to feel my strength. They encouraged me to use my voice.

We matter. We are worthy of love. We deserve to be happy.

We need our successes to be celebrated.

Stephanie George is a mom of four, stepmom of two, and lives in Jarvis, Ontario. She is an Indigenous midwife and international board certified lactation consultant and can be found at @mytimeatlast on Twitter and Instagram.

RECOVERY IS NOT PERFECTION

Alana Oikonen

WHEN I BROUGHT HOME MY first child, I brought home something else, too.

I remember how at first, my husband and I held our baby girl almost all the time. She slept in our arms, and we took three-hour shifts holding her through the night because that just somehow seemed like the right choice. She was so small, so vulnerable. How could we possibly let her go?

We fumbled our way through the first few months, as all parents do. I struggled to establish a breast milk supply via pumping when we were unable to breastfeed the *traditional* way. We finally figured out how to get our baby to sleep in a bassinet and not our arms.

Somewhere in these first few months, the other thing I brought home with me after my daughter's birth started to creep into my life.

I became irritable and anxious. I was borderline obsessive about pumping enough milk to feed my daughter, completely determined to not give her any more formula. I was that woman who literally cried over spilled milk when I dropped a bottle full of freshly expressed milk on the floor. I got snappy and easily frustrated. I hated when my husband seemed to be able to do things I couldn't. *Why didn't the baby cry when he changed her diaper? Why would she settle down to sleep with him, but not me?* All of these negative emotions led to some pretty ridiculous arguments, after which I would storm off and cry alone in the bedroom.

Crying became a norm—for the baby and for me. I pumped milk for hours every day. Often I sat at my pumping station, my daughter in her little bouncy chair and me, pumping for 45 minutes while she screamed the whole time. I would try talking to her, and rocking the chair with my foot—all to no avail.

I had several days where I felt like I was about to lose it—as in completely lose my mind and do something I would regret. I'd end up calling my husband, in tears, begging him to come home and take the baby for me because I just couldn't deal with one more minute of being stuck at home, alone, in the dead of winter with a baby who obviously (in my mind) hated me.

Perhaps you're reading this and thinking, *Wow, what a horrible mother.* Or maybe you're thinking, *I felt that way too.* Perhaps you might even be thinking, *That woman sounds like she's mentally ill.* That last piece, that's the truth. I was ill. When I'd gone home after the birth of my daughter, I had brought home a baby, and I had also brought home postpartum depression and anxiety. I just didn't know it yet.

I have to admit, I am a bit embarrassed to say that I didn't recognize my own illness. I have a master's degree. I work in mental health. I was completely aware that postpartum depression was a possibility and was never in denial about the fact that it could happen to me. Except when it did happen, it was nothing like I thought it would be.

It crept up on me: slowly, insidiously. The progression of fine, to slightly stressed, to stressed and tired, to not really functioning well in my daily life was so slow it all just seemed...normal. As if this was what parenting was; a horrible time of self-doubt, frustration, depression and panic, except no one ever warned me. It was a horrible secret everyone was keeping from first-time parents.

I also thought postpartum depression would be more...depressing. That I would be stuck on a couch, with no motivation to do anything and crying at the drop of a hat Instead, I was so frustrated and angry. Everything irritated me. I wanted help with the baby, but when my husband could do things easily and I couldn't I just hated him and I hated myself.

My mother moved in with us around this time, from halfway across the country. She was the first person to say something to me and suggest I might not be well. I just snapped at her and said I was fine. Because isn't that what you do?

Of course she was right. I wasn't fine. After her words had a couple days to sink in, I was able to admit the truth to myself. I was coming apart at the seams, and I needed help. I made a personal decision to talk to the doctor at my daughter's next check-up.

At the four-month check-up, the doctor who saw us was not my regular doctor. She was someone I had never met before, or even seen at the office. I knew going into the appointment that I was still not feeling well. Things were not getting better. My anxiety about producing enough breast milk was incredibly high. I was barely making it through the day. I often yelled and lost my temper, me, a person who had once described themself as having infinite patience. One of my regular clients at work calls me Smiley, but I certainly wasn't smiling much anymore.

The doctor did a perfectly good job of checking out my equally perfect, healthy baby. What she didn't do was ask me anything about how I was doing.

I was sitting there, in one of those completely uncomfortable plastic chairs, holding my chubby squirmy baby and waiting. Waiting for the moment when she was going to ask me about my mental health (which my regular doctor had done at our previous two-month check-up). The words were swirling around in my head, dancing on the tip of my tongue, just waiting to pour out. But she never asked. And I never told.

Instead, I sat there realizing this was the end of the appointment, and she wasn't going to ask and I had that feeling, that weighty feeling of knowing I should say something, but I couldn't. The words weren't just caught in my throat, they were caught in my brain. They were trapped in the mass of chaotic thoughts I had about myself and my situation: that I was not a good mother, that I should be able to make myself feel better, that this would just go away if only I worked harder to think positive, that this doctor would judge me horribly for admitting I sometimes got so angry at my baby I yelled at her, that I felt inadequate and incompetent, and that I would never get it together.

I don't remember leaving the doctor's office. To be honest, a lot of my memories of those early months with my daughter are kind of patchy, or missing altogether—like a blurry photograph where you can barely make out what's happening and certainly can't see any of the details.

I do remember having a conversation with myself about how I needed to try harder, how I needed to be more positive. I was smart, educated, had support, had a nice home and enough money to get out of the house and do things with my baby. I could fix this.

I couldn't fix it. It got worse. It got scary.

I started to have intrusive thoughts. I thought about how useless I was and how I should just leave and never come back. I thought about hurting my baby. I thought about hurting myself.

The next doctor's visit was the six-month baby check-up.

Before that appointment, I did one of the best and bravest things I have ever done. I told my mom I needed to ask for help, that I should have already asked for help, but I hadn't. I had her come to my appointment with me to make sure I got the words out. "I am not well. I need help."

I got them out.

Having my mom there and my regular doctor to talk to took that lump out of my throat and stilled some of the chaos in my mind. But it was still hard to say the words. It was hard to admit what felt like failure.

The first step was the hardest, which is a somewhat trite phrase that's used to talk about many types of journeys—but it's true. Finally telling someone, a professional outside my family, was a huge step. It was the first step to recovery and finding myself again.

If you are reading these words and seeing yourself in them—I wish I could tell you my journey after seeing the doctor was easy, but I can't. My daughter is six years old now. I had another baby after my daughter and went through perinatal mental health issues all over again, but worse (if you can believe it). I have come to the difficult but important conclusion that I will live with depression and anxiety for the rest of my life.

Recovery from any mental health issue involves many factors. It's about building resources and tools to help yourself. For me, I used a peer support group, medication, exercise, and a lot of self-compassion. I learned to re-evaluate my expectations for myself and for my children. I let go of some things I had previously thought were important because they were causing me too much stress and anxiety. I started asking for help.

I was able, over time, to be thankful for that help, not jealous and insecure. I learned that being vulnerable and talking openly with my husband, my mother, and other close supportive people about my struggles was not a weakness—it was brave and a true sign of strength. I learned to recognize the signs of when I was starting to get overwhelmed and began asking for help before I exploded. I still miss the cues sometimes. I still yell at my kids and then regret it later. Recovery is not perfection.

When we bring a baby home from the hospital, we expect to bring joy and happiness home with us. If we are realistic, we know that our lives are about to change and that things will be hard. Some of us, however, bring something a little extra home with us in the form of a perinatal mental health issue. If you or anyone you know is experiencing a perinatal mental health issue, know that you can reach out for help. You are not a bad mother, or a bad person. You are ill. And just like you would see a doctor for any other illness, you can see a doctor for this as well. You are not alone. With help from health care professionals, family, and other community support, you can recover.

Alana Oikonen is the mother of two sweet and spunky girls and lives in Prince George, British Columbia. She has a masters degree in occupational therapy and has spent her entire career specializing as a mental health OT. She is currently working toward becoming a certified perinatal mental health specialist. She can be found on Instagram @alanaoikonen

PSYCHOTHERAPY AND PERINATAL MENTAL HEALTH

Ryan J Van Lieshout, Donya Merza, and Erika Haber-Evans

A VARIETY OF EVIDENCE-BASED PSYCHOTHERAPY can be used to effectively treat perinatal depression and anxiety. The best outcomes are achieved when women have easy access to psychotherapies delivered by skilled therapists with whom they develop a good therapeutic relationship. Under these conditions, most women who engage in psychotherapy improve and become the mothers they all aim to be.

What is Psychotherapy?

Talk therapy or psychotherapy refers to the many ways that speaking with another person can help with psychological/psychiatric problems, as well as a range of other difficulties that do not exceed diagnostic thresholds for formal psychiatric diagnoses. Psychotherapy has long provided people with a way to express their personal experiences and help them conceive new ways of seeing themselves and their lives by helping them shift their thinking, feelings, and behaviour. The earliest forms of psychotherapy likely emerged in ancient Greece, pre-dating the advent of Judaism and Christianity.

Answers to the question of how and why psychotherapy works are as varied as the unique individuals who undertake it. It is generally thought that it helps give the individual someone to explore their problems with confidentially, enabling them to see themselves and their environments in new ways, and then move forward toward possible solutions. When successful, psychotherapy can help reduce the severity of troubling thoughts and/or emotional states, or even eliminate them so that one can function in the way that they want. Research suggests that up to 75-80% of people who enter into psychotherapy show at least some benefit from it.

Psychotherapy and Perinatal Mental Health

In the perinatal period, psychotherapy is most commonly used to help women overcome difficulties with depression (i.e., low mood), worry and anxiety, interpersonal problems, and the transition to motherhood. It can be delivered in individual format, in couples, or in groups. Not surprisingly, up to 90% prefer psychotherapy over medications because of concerns about the potential impact of pharmacotherapy on their fetus/infant.

While the different types of psychotherapy differ in the theories they are based on, most are about equally effective for depression when delivered by trained therapists. Psychotherapies are often classified as short or long-term, with short-term therapies ranging from 1-15 sessions, and longer-term treatments lasting months to years. Single sessions last 45-60 minutes, and most women who are treated successfully feel better in about six to 12 sessions (half improve after eight). Over half of women who receive a full-course of CBT (for perinatal depression or anxiety) or IPT (for depression) will have their symptoms completely resolve (i.e., remit). An additional 25% will experience substantial improvement.

The choice of which treatment is ideal for perinatal depression and anxiety should be guided by the severity of a mother's illness, one's previous response to treatment, and their preferences. Psychotherapy is recommended by clinical practice guidelines as the first formal treatment for perinatal depression. However, those with more severe illness (or those who cannot access psychotherapy) should consider medications as their benefits can outweigh their drawbacks. However, women who take medications can also benefit from psychotherapy since the combination may be more effective than either alone.

Types of Psychotherapy

The most commonly used psychotherapies in the perinatal period include cognitive behavioural therapy (CBT), interpersonal psychotherapy (IPT), and psychodynamic psychotherapy. These are delivered by physicians, psychologists, social workers, nurses, and/or other registered psychotherapists.

CBT helps individuals recognize and change the types of negative thought (cognitive) patterns and maladaptive behaviours that lead to depression and/or anxiety. In the perinatal period, these can include thoughts that one is (or will be) a bad mother, or uncontrollable worry about their baby's health and development, as well as avoiding activities that are typically pleasurable, including social contact or self-care. CBT is the most effective type of psychotherapy for perinatal anxiety.

IPT is another short-term treatment and helps people understand the interpersonal issues that contribute to their depression, and aids them in learning more adaptive ways to express emotions and communicate with others. Perinatally these frequently involve struggles with the loss of old roles (e.g., as fun, as a professional) and freedoms and adapting to new roles/routines.

Psychodynamic psychotherapy suggests that our behaviour and well-being is affected by our past (often childhood) experiences and that the resultant patterns of thoughts (which are thought to be 'unconscious' or outside of our awareness) and feelings affect our moods. It aims to improve self-awareness through self-exploration and expression of emotion, so that our past (and unresolved) difficulties no longer affect us as much in our current life.

Emerging evidence from our research group and others suggests that the benefits of psychotherapy undertaken during pregnancy and/or the postpartum period may occur for both mothers and their offspring. This is yet another reason for healthcare systems to make psychotherapy immediately available to all mothers with depression and/or anxiety who need it.

When Should Psychotherapy Be Used?

Before starting treatment with psychotherapy, it can be helpful to understand how it fits into recommended treatment pathways. For most perinatal women (those with mild to moderate depression and/or anxiety), psychosocial tools should be used as a first step. This includes receiving education about perinatal depression and anxiety, reading self-help books (e.g., Mind Over Mood), utilizing online self-help, and engaging in proper nutrition, exercise, sleep, time for oneself, and using supports.

If problems persist despite the use of these techniques, formal psychotherapy (e.g., CBT, IPT) is a recommended next step. Medications are considered after psychotherapy in treatment recommendations, but are often prescribed after the first step because psychotherapy can be challenging to access in many settings.

Finding a Therapist and Succeeding in Therapy

There are many excellent therapists who can help women recover from perinatal depression and/or anxiety. While they do not necessarily have to specialize in perinatal mental heath, there are some advantages to working with someone with specialized expertise.

However, finding a good, experienced therapist can be a challenge. In the setting of universal healthcare (i.e., in Canada), finding a publicly-funded therapist is difficult as they are generally restricted to physicians and mental health counsellors in hospitals or other funded programs. There is often more choice when it comes to private therapists (who are paid out-of-pocket or using insurance benefits), the large supply can make it a challenge to identify who might be best.

One place to start is to ask for a recommendation from your family doctor, a nurse, or community mental health worker. Leaders of spiritual or religious organizations, mental health associations, and self-help and support groups can also provide the names of therapists who could be helpful.

When you do reach out to a therapist, it can be helpful to interview them to see if they are a good fit for you. Asking questions about their education and professional training, the number of years of experience they have, any specialized perinatal training or expertise, and the type(s) of therapy they can deliver will help. You should also find out how many sessions they think will be needed, how much the treatment will cost, and if their services are eligible for insurance coverage.

The therapeutic relationship is essential to good outcomes in psychotherapy, so the act of interviewing potential therapists can be the first opportunity to see how you feel when you communicate with this person. The importance of taking this step cannot be overstated! Finally, you will want to know their policies around things like missed appointments, contact between sessions, and rescheduling.

Once you have selected a therapist, you can increase the likelihood of success by answering the following questions: *How would I like to be different by the end of therapy? What do I want to see change?* These can relate to changes at home, at work, and in relationships, as well as which symptoms or other problems you would like to see improve.

During therapy, one can maximize effectiveness by being open and honest. In therapy, any act of sharing your thoughts or feelings only serves to deepen the therapeutic bond and provide more 'grist for the mill'. Completing any homework that is assigned will also lead to better outcomes—psychotherapy is very much about learning new ways of thinking and acting, and so practice is essential. If you have the time, you can also ask if there are any supplementary materials that could benefit you (readings, workbooks, etc) and complete those as well.

If things are not improving, do not hesitate to raise these concerns with your therapist. Mentioning this can help them to optimize your treatment and make additional recommendations. In some cases, you may choose to end therapy early or switch therapists. Some great therapists are simply not a great fit for everyone, and they understand that.

A number of different types of psychotherapy can effectively treat perinatal depression and anxiety, but the best outcomes are obtained when women have easy access to skilled therapists who deliver evidence-based psychotherapies. Since relatively low numbers of women are able to obtain psychotherapy easily, it is vital that researchers and funders develop innovative approaches to increasing access so that women can recover from perinatal depression and anxiety and become the mothers they all strive to be.

Dr. Van Lieshout is the Canada Research Chair in the Perinatal Programming of Mental Disorders and a perinatal psychiatrist at McMaster University. Ms. Merza is a student in the Neuroscience Graduate Program at McMaster. Ms. Haber-Evans is a registered psychotherapist and Assistant Professor in the Department of Psychiatry and Behavioural Neurosciences at McMaster University. She and Dr. Van Lieshout are co-directors of Elle Psychotherapy (elletherapy.ca).

RIBBONS OF LOVE AND PANIC

Christina DeRoche

I CHOSE PARENTHOOD, BUT I did not choose the outcome post my babies being born.

Theoretically, I should have had a supportive birth process. I chose to be followed by midwives because of their support and detailed approach to maternal care. I had a supportive husband who helped me whenever I asked. And we had some close family around and friends who helped me navigate pregnancy and post pregnancy. The messages I received were that pregnancy was natural and postpartum would be fine.

Having babies should be easy. You'll bounce back in no time.

I was told I was a happy and lively person so I would be fine with a new baby.

They were wrong. Dead wrong.

I did not bounce back. My mind did not bounce back; it sunk. It was a dark time post each of my births. The second was the darkest for me.

Anthony was a colicky baby and he pushed me to the brink. I had problems breastfeeding him, and at a week postpartum, with my doula at my side late at night, I made the decision to formula feed.

Colic would haunt us for almost seven months. Nothing was helping the colic, and I was getting no sleep. Throughout the time of arriving home and my whole time with him at home, I was panicked. I would panic leaving the house, or with him screaming on our walks. I could not relax, ever. I worried about him feeling pain and screaming or fussing while I was out shopping.

I slept horribly because of it, and my relationship with my four-year-old daughter was strained. I could not connect with her, the little connection I did have. My partner had no clue how to help me. If he tried to help, I would panic that he was doing the wrong thing.

At six months postpartum when I began to have intrusive thoughts of dropping my baby, or hurting him unintentionally, I went to see my doctor. I was told I was suffering from postpartum anxiety and verging on psychosis. The combination of being overwhelmed, sleep deprived, and whatever else, was pushing my mental health to the brink. I was relieved and crying in his office.

I decided to take one more month than planned for maternity leave. That month, I decided, would be dedicated to getting help.

My doctor told me it would be better for me to seek out private services rather than refer me to publicly funded social work services. "It would be too long of a wait," he said. So I set out to find a private professional to help me within the confines of what my insurance would be willing to pay. I searched google for a list of providers in the area. I found a few, but they all cost the same amount, around $150 per hour.

I found a social worker but could only afford two sessions. Knowing this, she provided me with as many tools as she could before I stopped seeing her. I practiced what I learned and began to focus on little aspects I could control and worked on talking myself down when panic struck. I focused on my health, ate better, began exercising, and even got out and socialized a little more. I decided to go back to work nine months postpartum and that helped.

I started to feel better but anger became my new emotion. I was angry that my midwives did not see the signs of perinatal mental illness. I was angry that no one in fact saw the signs. I had heard of postpartum depression but why wasn't anyone talking about postpartum anxiety?

Why was it so difficult to find resources to help me through postpartum anxiety that also cost a small fortune? How the hell did other women get through it, especially those with no support or resources?

This anger fuels my new passion—fighting and researching practical ways of helping women and their partners through the maze of perinatal mental health. Let's face it, having a baby does not mean you are mentally prepared for the flood of emotions and demands that will be placed on you. So how in the world are you supposed to know when you have a postpartum mental illness? Is not the whole period of postpartum just one big mental health need? I think so. My anger has me questioning the health care system and I am now a perinatal mental health advocate.

I will make a difference.

Christina DeRoche is mom to Alessandra and Anthony and the Research Manager at Canadore College in Ontario. She is an advocate for family well-being and community-based needs research. Her current research and work focus is on creating community and applied research solutions for women and men experiencing perinatal mental health issues. Connect with Christina on Twitter @CVDeRoche

HYPERVIGILANT

Kiersta Hazlett

I WAS ABOUT FOUR MONTHS pregnant. I was sitting in my car, thinking about what I wanted to eat for lunch. I really wanted a sandwich—like a delicious deli sandwich full of yummy meat, cheese, and vegetables. Finally feeling like I had more energy and an appetite, I was so excited to go to this local deli that made the best sandwiches.

I don't think I can remember a sandwich tasting so good, but as I inhaled my second-to-last bite, it dawned on me—*I wasn't supposed to eat deli meat!* Deli meat had a higher risk of being contaminated with bacteria. I put my sandwich down and started googling everything I could about it. *What are the rates of contamination in salami and prosciutto? What are the risks of listeria infection to a fetus?* I started looking at the current meat recalls and researched what to do if you've eaten contaminated meat while pregnant.

Then came the guilt.

I should have known. How could I be so stupid? I'm going to be a horrible mother if I can't even keep my baby safe now. How can I possibly go back to work and face my co-workers? How could I have let this happen? People will think I'm an idiot! What kind of nurse does this? I literally teach "getting ready for baby" classes. How am I even competent enough to do that!?

At the time, I was a nurse working in the area of reproductive health and had been experiencing lots of thoughts that I brushed off as just worries. I kept telling myself it was normal to worry because pregnancy was such a major life change. I had been a worrier my entire life. But this was different—the thoughts and negative voice in my head were really intense. From that point on, they became almost constant.

After going through a miscarriage just a few months before, I was really concerned about losing this pregnancy as well. I worried about everything—especially doing something that could harm my baby. I made life difficult for those around me with my constant fretting—and relationships that were already challenging became more strained.

Even though I was always worried, my pregnancy was healthy and uneventful. I ended up needing to be induced at 42 weeks. As labour progressed, my baby became distressed, and I ended up needing an emergency C-section. It was at this point that things really started to get worse. I found it incredibly hard to sleep while in the hospital and was asked by my obstetrician to be discharged early because they needed the bed for other patients.

Before going home, I asked to see the lactation consultant because I wanted to make sure breastfeeding was going well. I knew the consultant because of some work we had done together and she told me I should know what to do. She was surprised I had questions. This really hit me hard at a vulnerable time. Yes, I am a nurse and I have a lot of education about breastfeeding, but at this point I had never done it myself. Her comment was enough to make me doubt myself and any ounce of confidence I had about this going well.

We were discharged home and within 24 hours admitted back in through the emergency room because my new baby was dehydrated. We had a full work-up done on her, including a spinal tap to check for infection and a catheter to collect a urine sample, as well as bloodwork. It was horrible having her go through all of that, but I knew bringing her in was the right thing to do.

My baby started on an IV and we began to supplement her with formula. I spent about eight hours in the ER, unable to rest and sleep. I was so worried about breastfeeding but wasn't allowed to breastfeed her until they felt she was stable. I asked if I could pump to help maintain my supply but the only pump available was up on the postpartum floor. No one could bring it down to me, and no one was able to help me up with a wheelchair, so I had to walk up to the fourth floor, three days post my C-section in pain and exhausted, while my husband stayed with our baby.

When I got to the floor, no one knew how to handle my request. I was given a spot in the corner of the back of the nurses station, with no privacy, to pump. It was humiliating and excruciating. We eventually were admitted to the pediatric floor and I was permitted to stay with my baby. I was given a pump and privacy and started to feel better knowing we weren't displaced. I wanted to start to breastfeed her more as I knew my milk was coming in and that we'd hopefully get off to a better start. But the orders were strict—we had to top her off with a lot of formula after feeding. This made it hard to feed her on demand because she would sleep so long in between feeds.

My worries about being able to breastfeed exclusively continued throughout our entire stay. We were discharged without any direction on how to wean off the formula or who to go to for help. Suffice it to say, my confidence was lost and I felt so defeated. My goal was to breastfeed, and the pressure I had put on myself to be successful at it was intense.

Once home, I reached out for support in the community with breastfeeding as my daughter was now having so much trouble latching. I decided to switch to bottle feeding with expressed milk and formula combined. It helped ease the amount of work and time that went into feeding but not my guilt.

Through all of this I remember being very weepy and emotional. I would openly share how stressed I was and how heavy this all felt, but not a single health care provider that I came in contact with assessed how I was doing—not during my pregnancy, not while in the hospital, and not postpartum. With each hurdle I encountered, my mental strength eroded. I wished someone would have asked how I was doing so that I could feel like I mattered too, that I wasn't just this vessel that brought this baby into this world and that was left to struggle while the focus of care was only on the baby, and to have that relief knowing that there was something up with me medically, not that this was some character flaw. I felt so guilty at the time thinking about my own needs. *What kind of mother would want anything but her baby to be okay?* If I was provided with the support I needed during this time, I think it would have made a lot of difference in my own outcome, and in the long-term health and wellbeing of my daughter as well.

Family members didn't seem to get it either with the exception of my parents. I remember being in the bathroom of a restaurant changing my baby's diaper, crying because I was so exhausted, in so much pain, but made to attend this event for a family member two weeks after giving birth. My then mother-in-law walked in and saw me crying. Instead of offering comfort or even help with my baby, I was told to stop crying—and that I wasn't the first woman to have a baby. It was yet another shot to my already non-existent confidence. One place where I found consistent acceptance and support was with my friends. It really was the only thing that made me smile. Just getting together once a week to vent about how challenging it was to be a new mom would help shift my mood and give me hope that we can do this together.

I started to develop symptoms of depression. I compare having both anxiety and depression at the same time as that weird state between being asleep and awake—you're conscious and aware of these terrifying thoughts but paralyzed to act on anything. At my worst point, I would lie awake most of the night, staring at the ceiling with this awful pit in my stomach and heaviness on my chest. During the day, I'd sit in the dark with no noise. I'd only get up to feed my baby and do what I needed to in order to care for her. I stopped eating, stopped doing anything to care for myself. I felt nauseous, heavy, and in a constant state of fogginess.

My most pivotal turning point was when I moved in with my parents while my then-husband went away on a trip with his friend. I had begged him not to go—not to leave me alone with our baby while I was feeling this way. He told me I was being selfish and that I wasn't thinking of him. I told him I wanted to die—that I wanted to leave and never come back. I didn't trust myself to be alone with her because, by this point, I was having intrusive thoughts about harming her. He blew me off as being dramatic instead of thinking that I needed support to get better.

Looking back on this time, moving in with my parents was the best thing I could have done. It gave them the chance to see how I was really doing and for me to feel safe telling them. My mom shared with me that she, too, had some intrusive thoughts about me after she had given birth. She encouraged me to make an appointment with my family doctor and even came with me to that first appointment.

My appointment with my family doctor was fairly straight forward —my mom did a lot of the talking, telling him how I was not acting like myself, while I sat there and cried. I told him about feeling worried and not being able to do much. He agreed that I was likely anxious and depressed and gave me a prescription for an antidepressant. He didn't probe much. I remember feeling like, *That's it?* He never asked if I was having intrusive thoughts, or if I was thinking of harming myself. I definitely didn't have the courage to come out and say it myself.

At this point, I truly believed that everyone would be better off without me. I was a burden because I couldn't take care of myself or my baby.

But I hadn't worked out a plan of how I wanted to end my life. I was scared and didn't actually want to die. It was so hard to struggle with those feelings. I wished I had been asked more about them. I wished someone had told me that I never was a burden, that I had a legitimate medical need.

My family doctor suggested I come back in six to eight weeks to see how the medication was working but didn't refer me to therapy or counselling. I wasn't able to advocate for myself much at this point, so the only step I took was to begin taking the medication.

Within a few weeks, I started to feel better. I can remember the pressure in my chest eased off first, and then I started to be able to sleep a little better. Slowly, over a few more weeks, I was worrying less and able to function more and more. I felt like doing things to show myself some self-care like taking a shower and doing my hair, making sure I ate and drank water, going for a walk, or getting together with friends.

Since the birth of my first child, I have had two other children and managed to keep my anxiety and depression managed with medication and connected with counsellors when I felt I really needed it, especially around times of exceptional stress. Something I've learned during this time is that even though it is possible to manage anxiety and prevent depression from returning with the right medication and support, it is something that will always be part of me. It is also something that I have to take full control over and work at on my own, with a support team behind me.

During my darkest times, I wasn't sure how I was ever going to feel better again. But as things improved, I became more and more aware of the fact that others were struggling like I was. I made a promise to myself that I would use my experience to help normalize getting help for others. My practice now is focused on supporting families prenatally through early childhood and often involves helping parents become more informed about perinatal mental illness, treatments, and supports while helping them access care in their community or beyond if needed. The health of our families depends on it, now more than ever.

Kiersta Hazlett is a mom of three and lives in Barrie, Ontario. She is a public health nurse and works with families in the Healthy Babies Healthy Children program. Connect with Kiersta on Instagram @kiersta10

IT'S OKAY TO FALL APART

Morag Wehrle

The midwife who greeted us for our very first appointment was warm and welcoming, and seemed almost as thrilled for our first baby as we were. We chatted easily as she took my blood pressure and made a copy of my health card.

"Has anyone in your family ever experienced postpartum depression?" she asked.

"Not that I know of," I said breezily.

We talked briefly about what postpartum depression (PPD) was. I listened carefully and made notes in the little book I had bought just for these appointments. Looking at this list of signs and symptoms, I felt secure. I felt prepared. I felt armed with knowledge.

I also felt healthy and strong. I did yoga and aquafit and shopped excitedly for tiny baby clothes. I read books about labour and birthing. I daydreamed about the beautiful ease of our long summer days together.

When things didn't turn out the way I'd expected, I told myself I was a failure.

Like most women, I had assumed breastfeeding would come easily. But it did not. It was excruciatingly painful. When I pumped around the clock in an attempt to increase my supply, I would gather depressingly tiny amounts of milk, as though I were trying to wring water from a sponge that had lain in the sun. My dreams of lying curled with my baby, drifting on a wave of bliss as she cuddled close to my heart, began to seem both cruel and ridiculous. I took this burden on, internalized it so thoroughly I didn't even see what I was doing. And with it, I set myself up to fall short of every expectation I had for myself.

The first time I gave my daughter a bottle of formula in public, a stranger approached me to ask me why I wasn't breastfeeding. "It's better for the baby and it will help you lose the weight!" she said brightly, and then recoiled in horror when I burst into tears.

I'm a calm person, I thought. *Tantrums won't happen to me because I'll be so loving and understanding*. And then there I was, more exhausted than I had ever been in my entire life, in a body that didn't feel like mine any more. There I was, whisper-screaming at my baby in the middle of the night because he refused to sleep, and I no longer knew what day it was. And instead of being able to meet myself with compassion, I took the blame. I looked at myself in the mirror night after night and said, "You are a terrible mother." I cried and swore I would do better, except I didn't know how to do better. And I blamed myself for that, too.

One day I was out walking with my baby who had recently decided at three months old that he would only nap in his stroller. I felt utterly drained. I had had a difficult, miserable pregnancy, and unlike my first child, who was now two and a half, my son did not seem to need sleep. My legs felt as though they were cast from lead. I had left my husband and daughter at home and I was pushing my blanket-wrapped baby along, watching his fluttering eyelids, willing him to finally give in.

I pushed him down the hill and towards the bridge that crosses the Upper Levels Highway, a busy east-west connector that separates my residential neighbourhood from our high street. Halfway across the bridge, I slowed to a stop and then stood, staring down at the traffic zipping by below me. The smell of exhaust and the roar of the engines rose toward me as though from a great distance. I was still except for my right hand, which constantly rocked the stroller back and forth to keep my son peacefully asleep. I don't know how long I stood there, mesmerized by the monotony of the non-stop flow of movement before a small voice spoke calmly in the back of my mind.

I could put the parking brake on the stroller right here. He'd be fine. People would see what happened right away. He wouldn't even be alone for a minute or two. They'd find my husband's number in my phone. Everyone would move on, and they'd be better off, eventually.

I considered, seriously, what the voice was saying. *It made some good points*, I thought. It did not occur to me to be shocked or upset at what the voice had to say. It all seemed entirely reasonable. I did not realize that I had reached a point of crisis and that I desperately needed help. At some point, I simply turned and continued walking, pushing the stroller aimlessly past the same shops and restaurants I did every day, while those thoughts settled like a stone at the back of my mind. And later that night, when it did occur to me that perhaps these thoughts were a bad sign, I resolved that I must never, ever tell anyone about them. If I revealed myself in all my brokenness, I thought, they might take my children away from me. That I did not see the contradiction here—that I was thinking about taking myself away from my children, and convincing myself they would be better for it—says a lot about why it took me almost four years to break that vow of silence.

In our modern world, many of us live far from family. We are deprived of that in-born village so often touted as essential to the raising of children. We celebrate the culture of busyness, pitching our non-stop drive through work, exercise, and life as a point of pride, as a race to be won. This means our friends are often not available to help, if we could even bring ourselves to ask. We sell ourselves the value of relentless positivity. We tell ourselves to buck up, to meditate more, to be thankful. We point to social media as evidence that we are more connected, more networked, more integrated than ever before; and yet loneliness and isolation were reportedly at record levels among the general population even before the global coronavirus pandemic.

There is something unique about the isolation that new motherhood brings. At the moment that red-faced, slippery little bundle is placed on your chest, your old life is gone in an instant. The old *you* is gone in an instant. A baby is born—but so is a mother, a whole new persona you now have to get to know. You are expected to embrace this new identity completely and unreservedly, to bask in the beautifying light of motherhood, while dealing with all the details of postpartum reality for which you could not possibly be prepared.

Complete strangers ask if you had a *natural* birth. People eye your still-round belly and ask if you're due soon even as you're pushing a newborn in a stroller. Facebook friends you haven't spoken to since high school pop in to your message box, trying to sell you expensive subscriptions of shakes or vitamins or exercise videos *to lose the baby weight! and get your body back! We tell new mothers to enjoy every moment*, without acknowledging that some moments are just plain hard.

No one warns you that it's possible to be head over heels in love with this tiny being, knowing that you would do anything in your power to keep them happy and safe—while also feeling the shock, the loss, the *grief* of the massive shift in life you've just undergone. No one tells you that your health, your nurturing, your nourishment is as important as your baby's. No one tells you that it's okay to fall apart.

But I believe, more strongly than ever, that it is vitally important for us to normalize these conversations. I know about isolation, the feeling of being completely and utterly alone and adrift with my dark and awful thoughts. I know about self-judgment and endless self-recrimination. I know about trying to live up to some impossible ideal and believing in my heart that I was doomed to failure. And I know anger and resentment over knowing these things. I know longing and regret and wishing I could go back.

And I know that there is no going back, only forward; and I know that motherhood has turned me inside out, taken me apart, and put me back together stronger than I was before. In sharing our stories, we remind ourselves, and each other, that we are in this together.

Morag Wehrle is a mom of three from North Vancouver, British Columbia. She is writing a book based on her experience of prenatal and postpartum depression in the hopes that it may help even one person feel less alone and broken. You can find Morag on Instagram @rainydaymo

PRECIOUS MOMENTS

Debbie Fazio

I WAS 24 YEARS OLD and married to my high school sweetheart when I gave birth to our first baby girl. She was the first grandchild on both sides of our family as well as within our circle of friends, so I didn't benefit from experience or knowledge passed down to me. During a very short, 24-hour hospital stay, I received very little education or support from the staff and was sent home with no direction other than to follow-up with my obstetrician in six weeks.

The first six weeks were a huge struggle, especially with breastfeeding. I had heard the phrase "breast is best." However, my daughter had a very poor latch, which resulted in bleeding and cracked nipples, and I wasn't producing enough milk. At our six-week postpartum follow-up appointment, I spoke to the obstetrician about this, and he really didn't have much information to offer other than to suggest I supplement with formula in a bottle as our baby was losing some weight.

Over the next couple of months, my experience as a new mother became so unenjoyable. I had absolutely no help from the day my daughter was born as my husband had to return to work where he worked over 16-hour days, and our family and friends lived far away. I remember my husband chasing me around the house with our daughter who was so hungry, but the pain that I was feeling at the breast when she would feed was so excruciating. I remember looking down at her once, as she was feeding and her mouth was covered in my blood. No one told me about breastfeeding consultants, and no one told me about breastfeeding clinics. I just grinned and bared it until our four-month visit to our doctor when I broke down in the office crying. I will never forget the words the doctor said, "Then just stop." At this moment, I felt this huge weight lifted off of me. I felt like the biggest burden of breastfeeding my daughter had been taken away ,and I could finally breathe. We decided to move our daughter onto bottles and formula and life seemed so much calmer.

When my daughter was 10 months old, I discovered I was pregnant again, and we were so excited! Around the five-month mark, at a routine doctor's visit, the doctor couldn't get a heartbeat. He believed I may have lost the baby and immediately sent me to the hospital for my first ultrasound. When we were at the hospital, the staff doing the ultrasound thought we were there for a routine visit because I was so far along, and she didn't realize I wasn't aware that I was having twins when she casually told me how busy I was going to be when the *twins* arrived. I was in completed shock. I went from thinking my baby had died to *having twins*! My emotions were all over the place. I didn't know what to feel. For the next two months, I had many complications with my pregnancy, so I was put on bed rest at home and then in hospital.

I started to become very depressed.

I was in the hospital for over a month, during the Christmas season, away from my family and my 16-month-old daughter, all while watching other women come and go after having their own babies. Ultimately, the doctors decided that I should have a C-section at 32 weeks.

The babies were born at 3.7 pounds and 4.2 pounds. They were tiny. They didn't look like normal babies, and they were both rushed off into incubators in the neonatal intensive care unit (NICU). I wasn't able to touch my babies for three days or hold them for over a week as they fought for their lives.

The struggle of having to heal from a C-section, spend as much time with my babies as possible going back and forth from home to the hospital, all while still caring for my toddler was one of the most difficult things I have ever had to do in my life. Sadly, my husband had to go back to work after only a few days of the babies being born, and I still had no help from family. I ended up having to register my daughter for daycare for a few days a week while I was at the hospital, and I was so blessed that a neighbour who had a baby the same time as I had my first daughter offered to take her whenever she could—she was my saving grace and I never forgot that.

The babies spent just over a month in the hospital. During this time, the nurses were incredible. They taught me so many things about newborns and preemies and I was so thankful for their guidance and for the care of my babies. I wasn't one of the mothers who could stay at the hospital 24/7 as I was also trying to juggle caring for my toddler.

Leaving the babies in the hospital overnight while I went home was so difficult. I remember lying in bed crying, feeling sad, scared, worried, and disappointed in myself. Up until this time, I had been pumping as much milk as I could and the babies were being tube fed breastmilk and formula as they were too tiny to be at the breast.

One day, the NICU nurse told me the babies were strong enough to suck and asked if I wanted to try and latch them onto my breast. My heart started to pump so fast through my chest. On the one hand, I was so excited that the girls were strong enough to suck, but on the other hand, all those horrible feelings from my breastfeeding experience with my first daughter came flooding back.

I sat in the chair and lowered my shirt as I watched the nurse walk over to me. It felt like it was all happening in slow motion. She placed one of the babies in my arms. I reached for my breast and tried to latch my daughter. In that very moment that she tried to open her tiny little mouth, I broke down in tears and told the nurse I couldn't do it. The nurse was so kind. She quickly gave me a bottle, and we fed my daughter together. That nurse said something to me that I will never forget, "The most important rule is to feed the baby." Immediately, my anxiety and my fears started to ease.

Over the next few weeks, that nurse encouraged me, educated me, supported me, and truly cared. She was able to bring me to a place where I could breastfeed the babies when I wanted to and still bottle feed them when I couldn't. The pressure was off, and it felt incredible.

Once the babies came home, life with three children under two was definitely a challenge. People watching from the outside thought I had it all together, and to be honest so did I. Looking back on that first year, I can say I survived, but I did not enjoy it as much as I would have if I had had help. I recognize that not having the education and the support that I should have received affected my entire experience and my mental health and was never treated.

I didn't want that to happen to other moms so I created what was most lacking in my experience: a village. I put together a team of over thirty professionals that range from nurses to perinatal support workers, doulas and sleep consultants. Our team is focused on supporting and educating new and expecting families on pregnancy, birth and parenting. We offer physical, educational, and emotional support so that no parent ever has to feel like I did...alone.

There has always been a village to help raise our children but somewhere along the way, this changed. Somewhere in history, moms started to think they needed to do everything on their own and be supermoms, but this is not how it is supposed to be. The village I created helps to educate, mentor, coach, and guide new parents. We also listen to them, assess them, console them, support them, and be there for them. It's my honour that out of my own very difficult experience, I have created the village that so many parents need.

Debbie Fazio is a mother of three and lives in Hamilton, Ontario. She's a Parenting & Empowerment Coach and the founder and CEO of Precious Moments Babeez Inc. She is a Newborn Care Specialist, Happiest Baby instructor and a Board Certified Sleep Consultant who works with families around the globe. She is also the co-Founder and faculty for the Global Perinatal Support Worker (PNSW) Program Inc. in Canada (www.pnsw.org). You can find Debbie on Instagram @preciousmomentsbabeez

THE DAY I BROKE

Lori Waring

I REMEMBER THE DAY I broke.

I remember the day I couldn't take it anymore.

I remember the dark feelings and how they were taking over my mind despite every effort to try and remind myself that they were not a part of me—that they were not welcome and that they needed to leave.

I remember every scream and every tear from both me and my baby. I was not okay. And that meant that he would not be okay either. He needed me and I was broken. We both needed saving.

It's 2 p.m. on a Wednesday and I have been crying on the couch since my husband left for work at 6 a.m. This is my new normal. This is how I spend my days since I became a mother. I feel trapped. I feel lost. I feel alone, depressed, and terrified. And as I sit here looking at my beautiful baby, I feel nothing but regret.

What have I done? How could I have wanted this for my life? How will I ever be happy again?

A mother should love her child, and I feel none of that. My heart is shattered and so is my mind and body. I am not okay. I cannot let this go on any longer or I feel the worst could happen to us. So I search for something or someone who can help me.

I call a nurse at the local health unit and cry on the phone to her for over an hour. She is worried for me and connects me with the mental health crisis line. Again I cry to them, but this time in relief as I know that someone is going to help me get the help and support I need. This amazing lady on the other line gets it. She understands. She tells me it isn't my fault and that it is okay to feel the way I am feeling despite me being ashamed and terrified. She stays on the phone with me until I am comfortable hanging up and tells me to connect with my family doctor right away because I am being diagnosed with postpartum depression.

I have struggled with depression throughout my entire life. I am not sure if it stemmed from the emotional trauma I had faced when younger or the daily physical pain I experienced since I was a teenager, but regardless, this new type of depression was ten times more intense than anything I had ever felt before.

I am numb. I am exhausted.

I haven't smiled in over two months, and I want everything to end. It crosses my mind numerous times to just get up and run away, but I could never do that. Suicide is an option of escape, but I shook away that thought too. Most of the dark thoughts plaguing my mind are things that I cannot picture myself doing. But the thoughts are here, and the thoughts are real. They terrify me to my core and they need to be gone.

Now. They need to be gone now. They need to be gone before it is too late.

I hate the isolation I feel from being trapped at home all the time with a newborn. I hate how much I miss my old life. I hate my new obligations and how I am unable to uphold any of my old ones. This leaves me feeling worthless and selfish for wanting more.

Other people need me, and I am no longer able to be there for them. I have no idea how to take care of a baby and I am unable to take care of myself.

I hate that I hate being a mom.

How could I have put myself and my husband through so much pain over the years of infertility and not be happy when we finally got what we had always wanted? How can I not be satisfied? How can I not love the beautiful baby boy who clings to my arms? How can I resent him so much for how I am feeling? It is not his fault. This is my fault.

The thing I find with depression is that it magnifies every emotion that you are feeling but also provides a type of exhaustion that sleep just cannot fix. I try to sleep, I really do, but every time I try my anxiety skyrockets and I lay awake dreading the next feeding, or listening for a cry that I don't know how to calm. I dread the monotony of the coming day, wondering when it will ever end. I feel trapped and unsure of how I am going to be able to keep going.

I start taking anti-anxiety and antidepressant medication after seeing my family doctor but am told it will take six weeks for me to feel the full effect and more like myself again.

How can I survive that long? How much longer will I have to feel my heart race, listen to the dark thoughts in my head, feel the heat of the tears on my cheek and the rawness in my throat from all the screaming in pain?

As the weeks go by, I begin to feel a little more like myself again, or at least I am hoping that I am. My husband works from home some days, and during the days when he can't, my other family members come and stay with me.

I feel like I need a babysitter to prevent me from doing the unthinkable when no one is watching. This makes me feel worthless, and I doubt how I am ever going to be a good mother. The darkness inside me is winning, and I don't know what it is capable of.

As the Christmas break nears to an end and I realize my time of having a second set of hands is almost over, the darkness begins to grow even more powerful.

For the second time since the birth of my beautiful baby boy, I have to admit to myself and my husband that I am not okay. I go back to the doctor and meet with my nurse on a weekly basis. We make a solid plan that I need to be more honest with my feelings if I am ever going to learn to control them.

So begins a lot of self-reflection and some cognitive behavioural therapy.

I realize that I need to not be embarrassed or ashamed of how I am feeling—they are my feelings, and I am allowed to feel however I need to. I need to be more honest and speak up when I need something and most importantly, I need to take care of myself and remember that the person I was before I became a mom is still here. I just need to find her again. All moms can relate that even just making sure you have a shower every few days feels like such an accomplishment with a newborn. But to offer yourself even more self-care, you need to do more. So I make sure I go for a hike every day and I pick up some new hobbies. The time I have is minimal but I work it in when I can.

I start trying to replace my negative thoughts with new ones.

It's okay if you thought you were over it, but it hits you all over again. It's okay to fall apart even if you thought you were in control. You are not weak. Healing is messy, and there is no timeline for healing.

I start to feel a little better. A little more like me. A little more light in the darkness. I feel optimistic. I feel in control. I am doing everything I need to be doing to feel better.

I am taking my medication, I am eating healthy, and exercising daily. I am checking in with my nurse, doctor and therapist on a regular basis, and I have a wonderful group of moms who I connect with daily. We met through an online support group and their love and openness is just what I need to reassure myself that I am not alone.

But the negative thoughts always return.

What if while I am doing everything right, my life still crumbles around me? What if, despite my best intentions, I keep falling too close to the edge again? What if I am fighting my hardest, but the darkness is fighting even harder?

Time goes on. Progress is made, but two steps forward feels like a million steps in reverse most days.

I'm not the me I remember nor the me I want to be. I am lost—I am not in control.

It is so difficult to explain what is going on in my head when I don't even understand.

This is me. This is still me. Not the me I want to be, but the one that I keep coming back to. The one who cannot control her emotions. The one who doesn't see the good in things. The one who wants to sleep all day and just turn everything off and embrace the dark.

This battle is exhausting.

When my baby turns six months old, I convince myself that I am going to be better soon. I am through the rough patch and I am seeing clearer.

But I'm not.

By the time he is eight months old I have tried numerous different medications and convince myself that I will be better by the time his first birthday rolls around.

But I'm not.

I start seeing a different therapist, am referred to a psychiatrist and meet with a naturopath. With all this help, I am certain that I will be myself by the time I return to work the following month.

But I'm not.

Something is missing. Something is still wrong with me.

Every time I think I see the end in sight, it just moves further away. It is out of reach, and it is soul crushing. I have exhausted all resources, all ideas, and all referrals but nothing has worked. I am exhausted and sick of fighting a losing battle. I don't have the strength to keep going.

I have lost myself. And I have lost control. Control of my body. Control of my mind.

My mind wanders towards unsafe thoughts, often. My brain feels foggy from the constant battle of trying to find ways to get better. My body shakes to the point where I can't even hold onto a pencil because of the extreme daily anxiety. My eyes hurt from the fatigue and my head is dizzy from all the confusion.

When I can't sleep, I think about every bad moment that has happened in my life and obsess over the ones that lay ahead of me. And when I can sleep, I never want to wake up and I don't have the energy or desire to get out of bed in the morning.

I have lost over ten pounds. I feel like my body is giving up on me. It is slowly shutting down. I cry every day.

And as I sit here, day after day, wondering when I will be able to stop pretending that I am happy and actually feel real happiness again, I start to realize that day may never come.

It has been so long since I have been able to enjoy life. I'm not even sure what I used to enjoy about life before. Deep down, I know I used to be optimistic and positive, but not anymore. My happy memories are now clouded by sad ones. It's as if I have erased every good moment from my past. My brain has decided that I will now be living in misery for eternity and the hope that I once had for better times is just that—hope. Not real. Not obtainable.

I only see the bad, and I spiral even more.

If I can't figure out a way to find happiness, am I stuck below the surface trying to learn how to breathe on my own forever?

People want to help me, I know they do. But they can only do so much. They can hand me the tools and show me how to use them but, in the end, I am the one drowning.

If I cannot learn how to swim to the surface, am I destined to just lie on the bottom on my own forever?

Darkness is scary. Thoughts that are not my own are scary. Feeling alone is scary.

But the thing that is the scariest to me is the feeling of running out of time. Time to heal. Time to breathe. Time to win against my inner enemies.

I have tried everything—and I mean everything. to get better. I have researched and tried every type of therapy and remedy to get me away from the bad thoughts and feelings, but nothing has worked. And the more things I try, the more depressed I become. I should be better by now. I should have found something that worked for me. I should be happy.

But I'm not.

Now I'm angry and resentful.

Why can't anyone figure out what is wrong with me? Why can't I figure out how to be myself again?

The fear of going too far and not being able to return is overwhelming. It's not that I am suicidal, but I know I need a way out—away from the depression—away from the ongoing anxiety and daily panic attacks—away from the dark memories and losses that I faced throughout my life. I hope something bad will happen to me so that I can end up in the hospital and get away from it all for a while. While driving home one day, I think that if I get hurt then at least I can sleep away the exhaustion in peace for a while. I'm trying to imagine a different life filled with everything I enjoy and none of the pain I am feeling.

But that life does not exist.

I begin drinking throughout the day and night to try and shut down for a while. I become obsessed with tracking my mood and how it relates to the time of day, the foods I eat, the medication I take—searching for the tiny moments of good feelings—trying to see how I can recreate them over and over again.

When I watch my little guy play and laugh I find joy—I love him with all my heart. Why will those feelings not stay with me? *Why do they come and go so fast and then I end up sitting here with a fake smile on my face and my mind begins to wander to sad thoughts? Why can't the bits of happiness I find replace the depression? Why are these perfect moments masked by my uncontrollable anxiety and fear?*

My head hurts. My heart races. My body trembles and my jaw clenches.

It is simple. I am unwell. It is not my fault. But I am unwell.

But the solution is not so simple. Healing is not easy. There will always be scars, the pain will linger on and wounds will reopen often—even when you think they are healed.

I don't know where I find the strength, but somehow I do and decide to never give up.

I will not back down from this fight. I will keep pushing through. Each day is a new chance to be the best mom, wife, sister, daughter, and friend that I can be.

This is my story but this is not the end. And it is not the end of your story either. There are brighter days ahead.

Lori Waring is a mother of one and lives in Bradford, Ontario. Follow her journey on her blog at www.myinfertilityjourney966670578.wordpress.com.

FOREVER CHANGED

Jaime Charlebois

I HAVE WRITTEN AND REWRITTEN this story. It doesn't get easier to tell. Sixteen years later, I am still feeling raw and vulnerable.

This is my story—a story of how my body reacted to pregnancy and postpartum, how it failed me, mentally and physically, and how I was robbed of the mothering experience I had dreamed of my whole life.

My husband and I were living the dream. We were established in our careers, we had a home, and we had family around us. We were happy.

We had always talked about having two kids. When we conceived, I had been a nurse for three and a half years and my hubby had recently switched careers and landed his dream job as a firefighter in the city he was raised. We had been together for six years, married for three.

My best friend was three months pregnant at the time and we were excited.

My pregnancy started as any other, but around six weeks in, I started having severe nausea, dizziness, and vomiting, I was later diagnosed with Hyperemesis Gravidarum (HG). I have since learned that HG increases your risk of developing postpartum mood and anxiety disorders (PMADs). I was off work for ten weeks and lost 20 pounds—I was wasted and weak. My poor baby was nourished with toast, crackers, ginger ale and Gatorade. I was lucky that it passed around 20 weeks and I was able to resume work. For some women, it can occur throughout the entire pregnancy and result in hospitalization.

I was never screened or asked about my mental health in pregnancy or postpartum. I actually had so many risk factors that I now recognize because I have more knowledge about PMADs. I wish someone had prepared me.

I can honestly say my daughter's birth, as fast as it was (only five and a half hours), was the best part of our journey. The first three months postpartum were amazing and pretty easy. My hubby was a true partner, and we got into an early rhythm. Our daughter was happy and slept through the night. We both wondered why other people said the first three months were horrible. We must have cursed ourselves because then the floor fell out from under us.

At three months postpartum, I had my first major gallbladder attack. I woke up at 3 a.m. with back pain, sweating and shortness of breath, and then the back pain moved around to the front just below my chest. I thought I was having a heart attack.

I was pacing while we waited for the ambulance to come. They took me to the emergency room, and my hubby woke up our daughter and met me there. By the time the doctor saw me, the pain was gone. They ordered blood work and an ultrasound. I remember the nurse saying that I was probably having a gallbladder attack, but the ultrasound and bloodwork were inconclusive.

From that moment on, our daughter didn't sleep for more than 20-40 minutes at a time. I had planned to make all my own baby food, but I simply didn't have the time or energy. I continued to have gallbladder attacks for five more months until my surgery at eight months postpartum.

I became sleep deprived and extremely anxious. I bought books to figure out how to help my daughter sleep. I'd get into a depressive cycle when none of the techniques I tried worked until my hubby told me to just take the book back. As soon as I did, the depression subsided. This happened several more times.

I can't remember what came first, the anxiety or the complete change in our daughter's temperament, but it got really hard. I couldn't put her down, ever, without her screaming. She wanted me and only me, and this was very overwhelming. She was exclusively breastfed, which I wanted, but I had a huge milk supply. I wanted her to take a bottle so I could get breaks or so my hubby could help, but she never accepted a bottle (and we bought every one!). The ironic thing was when I was offered breaks, I couldn't take them. I'd become so anxious when I heard her cry, and I would swoop in to rescue her.

I started to isolate because our daughter was so difficult. If my hubby was at work, I went to my parents, in-laws or friend's house. I needed their support. I doubted every thought I had, every move I made, and every action I took. I started journalling and tracking my daughter's sleep—or lack thereof. I now know I had postpartum obsessive-compulsive disorder at this point. I was neurotic, and I started having intrusive thoughts that were horrifying and persistent.

Guilt, there was so much of it. I questioned everything, especially myself.

Things didn't settle until our daughter was about 18 months old. I didn't feel normal, hormonally, until I had completely weaned her from breastfeeding. By then it felt like a dark (weighted) blanket was lifted. I felt like myself again. Around that time, my friends were all talking about having baby number two. But my hubby and I both knew that we couldn't do it all again. We decided instead to stay happily married and nurture our little family. Our ordeal had taken a toll on our relationship.

People were outright rude about our decision to have only one child, but we have never regretted our decision. I joke that my master's degree was my second child. I had part of my thyroid out around four years postpartum and also joked that I couldn't have another baby because I didn't have many vestigial organs left. Honestly, I was traumatized by my postpartum experience. I had nightmares and flashbacks and couldn't fathom doing it all again.

I am a person who is comfortable with being open and honest. I told everyone about my struggles, doubts, and inadequacies. I didn't speak to a health-care practitioner because I wasn't overly depressed so I didn't really know there was anything wrong. I just thought it was me.

Due to the untreated nature of my PMADs, I'm forever changed. I do deal with mild to moderate anxiety that I have learned to cope with and manage. I have had Premenstrual Dysphoric Disorder since I had my daughter (more common after experiencing PMADs), and my hormones continue to be a challenge. Menopause should be fun!

My one piece of advice beyond the typical reach-out for help is to trust your own instincts. If something doesn't feel right, tell someone, get support. PMADs are treatable.

We need to prioritize women within the childbearing years because there is no health without mental health.

Jaime Charlebois is mom to Lauryn and lives in Barrie, Ontario. She is the co-founder and research director of the Canadian Perinatal

Mental Health Collaborative. She is also the perinatal mood disorder coordinator at Orillia Soldiers' Memorial Hospital and regional volunteer coordinator for Postpartum Support International.

GOOD ENOUGH

Sarah Cunningham

FOR AS LONG AS I can remember, I have wanted to be a mother. When I was younger, I loved playing with dolls, and as I got older, I took babysitting courses and cared for neighborhood children. When I was a teen, I coached youth, and now as an adult, I work with children of all ages. I love working with children, and I couldn't wait to have a child of my own.

My husband Kyle and I were both looking forward to starting our family, and neither of us could have imagined what our journey to parenthood would look like. After many months of trying to conceive with no success, we decided to seek medical advice.

I felt like I was being brushed off because I was young and healthy, but I knew something wasn't right. After many more months of getting the testing that I was pushing for, I was diagnosed with Polycystic Ovarian Syndrome (PCOS), a condition that was affecting my hormone levels and making it harder for me to get pregnant. Once I was diagnosed, we were referred to a fertility clinic and after three cycles of fertility medication, I finally got the positive pregnancy test we had been wishing for.

My entire pregnancy was smooth, and I felt amazing throughout. I felt so grateful and loved being pregnant. I assumed that I would love motherhood just as much. I remember I had a detailed birth plan: I wanted a drug-free, vaginal birth. I regularly saw my naturopath, did acupuncture, and had chiropractic adjustments to prepare my body. I practiced prenatal yoga, and I read all the books.

My water broke unassisted at home, which I thought was a great sign that my body was following all the usual steps. Within 24 hours, on my birthday, my daughter Leah was born via an unplanned C-section. As much as I had planned for the birth I wanted, the entire experience felt out of my control. It left me in a state of both physical and mental distress.

After only two nights in the hospital, we were sent home. I was in so much pain that I ended up sleeping on the couch, unable to make it into our bed. Leah cried non-stop no matter how much I tried to breastfeed, rock her, soothe her, and five days later we were readmitted to the hospital. My milk still had not come in and Leah was dehydrated, which explained why she was constantly crying.

I felt awful, like I had already failed my daughter. I felt that my body had failed—at trying to conceive, at giving birth, and now with breastfeeding too.

Nothing seemed to be going the way I had expected it to; I thought I would feel immense joy and unconditional love, but I couldn't stop crying. Leah was colicky and I was exhausted all the time. I felt anxious carrying her on the stairs or driving with her. I constantly stressed over whether she was getting enough to eat; I didn't want her to become dehydrated again. I couldn't understand how, after wanting a baby so badly, I just didn't feel happy.

At my six-week checkup, my obstetrician asked me how I was feeling. I mentioned that I cried often, didn't feel like myself, and was feeling more anxious than usual. She then asked, more like stated, "But it's not postpartum depression, right?" This confused me. At the time, I wasn't sure what was considered normal and what was seen as perinatal mental illness, so I wasn't sure if I should be asking for help. So I didn't. I said, "No, I guess it's not postpartum depression." Left untreated, my symptoms persisted and worsened.

I was four months postpartum when I realized I needed to do something about my mental health; something definitely wasn't right with how I was feeling. I was plagued with guilt. I felt that if I had postpartum depression, it somehow made me ungrateful for the baby we had wanted so badly. I booked an urgent appointment with my family doctor for the next day. I expressed my symptoms of rage, hopelessness, anxiety, and exhaustion—all uncharacteristic of me. I felt hopeful that I was finally admitting how I was feeling and that I would get the help I needed. It took so much bravery for me to come forward, but the only thing my doctor offered was to place me on a four-month waitlist to see a psychiatrist. I was crushed. I couldn't wait another four months.

As a last attempt, I sent an email to a private psychologist specializing in perinatal mental health whom I'd found by searching the Internet. If this connection didn't work out, I was ready to give up. I was exhausted trying to find the help I needed. Thankfully, we did connect, and I became a patient of Dr. Tanya Cotler right away. I could tell that she genuinely saw my pain and cared about my well-being. I saw her weekly for many months, driving almost an hour from my home to her office. Although private therapy was both costly and time consuming, for me, it was well worth the investment. I felt lucky to be able to afford it. Finding a health-care provider I could trust was a game changer for me; it was the defining moment of how the rest of my postpartum journey would play out.

While still in therapy, I asked for a referral to the Women's College Hospital Reproductive Life Stages Program, which I eventually started nine months postpartum. I was formally diagnosed with postpartum depression and postpartum anxiety, and with the psychiatrist there, I decided to add medication to my care plan. I was discharged three months later due to the fact that the program doesn't treat women past one year postpartum. My psychiatrist did offer to see me past the one-year mark, however I was returning to work full time and could no longer make the commute to downtown Toronto to attend appointments.

When I returned to work, a sense of routine and normalcy helped me settle. I started a new job, which I loved, and met new friends and coworkers who became my village of support. I thought I was coping fairly well and began weaning myself off my medication over the summer. I hadn't been doing therapy due to the time constraints of working full time. When the winter hit, I noticed my mood was worsening again and before long, the original symptoms of rage, depression, and anxiety were returning. I reached out to my family doctor for another psychiatrist referral. Then one month later, the COVID-19 pandemic hit, and I was laid off as my workplace was mandated to close.

My mood was still rapidly declining, and the frequency of my worst episodes were increasing. The waitlist to see a psychiatrist was almost a year long, so I reached out to my previous private psychologist and got back into therapy. It was virtual this time due to the pandemic, but I didn't mind. It was comforting to see a familiar face. A couple of months later, I got a call from my original psychiatrist referral. I had reached the six-month mark since being referred, and although it was still a year-long waitlist, they were willing to offer me a one-time phone call to do a medication consultation. I figured this would be a great option especially since I was under the care of a psychologist, and all I needed was a medication plan.

After a 20-minute phone call where I described some of my symptoms, the doctor pushed me to do further testing for bipolar, which didn't feel like the right fit to me. Although myself and my psychologist both respectfully disagreed with his tentative diagnosis, the doctor I spoke to on the phone would not prescribe anything without further testing. I am so grateful that with my psychologist's help, I was able to get an appointment with a psychiatrist in the perinatal program at Mount Sinai Hospital for a second opinion.

After a thorough consultation with the doctor at Mount Sinai, she confidently ruled out bipolar, agreed with my original diagnoses of postpartum depression and anxiety, and also added the diagnosis of Intermittent Explosive Disorder (IED). She believes the episodes I was having were a result of suppressed grief after losing my mother as a child, which resurfaced after the birth of my daughter. My body didn't have the opportunity as a child to learn to process these big emotions and this is how they were showing up.

She truly listened to my full story and got me on a proper medication plan, which seemed to be the final puzzle piece for me. This, combined with weekly therapy has made an incredible impact.

My daughter is now almost three, my mother died almost 20 years ago, and I am finally starting to properly work through my grief and trauma.

Before becoming a mother, I had heard of postpartum depression but had no idea how common it was. I hadn't considered that it would happen to me. I'm surprised that I wasn't screened during pregnancy or postpartum as I had so many risk factors: fertility struggles, traumatic birth experience, a colicky baby, sleep deprivation, and mental health struggles related to the loss of my own mother. I had no idea how intensely my grief would return after becoming a mother myself.

It took a lot of advocating for myself to get the help I needed, and I am so grateful to have such a wonderfully supportive husband. This journey caused some of our darkest times together, which definitely put stress on our relationship, but it has also brought us closer and ultimately given us our greatest gift: Leah.

I can finally say that I am truly enjoying motherhood and enjoying life. I am learning how to identify my own needs as I also navigate my daughter's. I'm far from perfect, but I feel like a good enough mother. This entire experience has made me want to make sure other moms know that it's okay to struggle, it's okay to need help, and that even though it may not feel like it—it really does get better with the right treatment.

Sarah Cunningham lives in Bowmanville, Ontario with her husband Kyle and their daughter Leah. She works with kids and families at Life Time Athletic. You can find Sarah on Instagram @sarcunningham_

FROM CRANKY MOMS TO WELL PARENTS

Dr. Jillian Satin and Dr. Samantha Waxman

As clinical psychologists, we were gaining confidence. Armed with PhDs, we each stepped into our careers in private practice feeling ready to contribute professionally, with typical bouts of imposter syndrome. Though we had not met each other yet, we shared the same passion for health psychology and had each taken an avid interest in perinatal mental health.

A few years later, we each entered the transition to motherhood. That transition was bumpy. We vividly remember the lack of sleep, the endless crying (thank you colic), the constant worry, and our sore changed bodies. It felt very, very lonely—both in terms of the actual time spent alone with baby, and also as if nobody understood our individual experience. We remember being awake in the middle of the night and feeling like we were the only people on the planet.

As psychologists with perinatal mental health training, we thought we had reasonable expectations of what motherhood might look like. We had worked with many postpartum clients. We had friends and siblings with kids, and we witnessed their evolutions. We thought we knew, but we did not. The transition was beyond what we could have imagined. Like so many mothers today, we thought it would be easier to get it right, to read a book (or ten) and know what to do. We quickly realized that you can educate yourself all you want, but you can't always get a baby to sleep, eat, and burp whenever you choose, even if you follow all the best advice.

We met on Canada Day 2014 at a mutual friend's house. Professionally, we automatically had something in common. Since we were both on maternity leave, we quickly learned that if you can carry on a conversation with someone relatively easily, then this person is now part of your circle. Someone to spend time with, to pass the hours, to vent, and to get advice from. We started to celebrate milestones and holidays together. On our first postpartum Halloween, Jill's son (a monkey) and Samantha's daughter (Olivia Newton-John, sweatband and all) played together. We participated in strollerfit classes, mommy groups, and play-dates—memories that solidify for us the importance of social support in the postpartum period. We frequently discussed the challenges associated with the postpartum period. We had felt competent and confident in our professional lives, yet we found ourselves dumbstruck by how unprepared and disoriented we felt in our new postpartum lives. It was at that time that we started dreaming of what we now call The Well Parents Centre.

Our professional purpose became clearer and we have been laser-focused ever since. Coincidentally, we had our second children three years later, only three weeks apart. Luckily for us, we were able to swap wardrobes so neither of us had to buy anything new for the babies (second kids!) and we found a built-in support system in each other every step of the way. Parents often seek reassurance and validation that their behaviours and choices are normal and reasonable, and it is so nice when you don't have to search for those answers on the Internet. During our parental leaves, we sought out further training and certification as perinatal mental health providers through Postpartum Support International. We pursued advanced training out of town; our first time away from our babies, which resulted in us going to bed at 8 p.m., though we planned on having a big night out to celebrate. We sat in parks and coffee shops and brainstormed ways to help other parents with this transition. Although the focus of our clinic never changed, we tested out a series of names. After a particularly exciting brainstorming session, we came up with the name "Two Cranky Moms" for our clinic and thought we were absolutely brilliant. Beaming with pride, we shared our lightbulb idea with our husbands who very quickly told us this was a terrible idea. We still like the name, so we've tucked it away for if we ever open a coffee shop for tired parents.

Through our own experience and through our privilege of speaking with many parents over the years, we have gained some insight into the postpartum period that we hope can make the transition easier for others. A benefit of developing a niche and seeing so many clients with similar issues is that themes emerge more clearly. In our work with postpartum clients, we often share these themes and insights. Clients remark that hearing these themes mirrored back to them provides the validation and normalization that they so needed. We hope the insights below help a reader.

First, parenthood is an adjustment, and it can be awkward and difficult. Think back to adolescence and going through puberty. The transition to becoming a mother is similar in its awkwardness. Reproductive psychiatrist Dr. Alexandra Sacks popularized the terms *matrescence* to describe this transition. Many women, particularly those with a strong need for achievement or control, can struggle with this clunky phase. The antidote? Self-compassion. Give yourself a minute to adjust, and be humble enough to ask for and accept help. If you think you *should* know what to do (e.g., how to bathe or feed baby, how to get baby to sleep), or that you *should* be able to manage on your own or with very little sleep, you will add suffering to what is already hard. We didn't think we would need to ask for help as new parents, but when we did seek the help of breastfeeding consultants and then sleep consultants, we were so happy we did. We thought parenting was supposed to be intuitive, but now we know that seeking parenting help in the form of coaching or online courses can be so valuable. There is no shame is not knowing, and there is power in learning.

Parents, and especially mothers, can feel a strong need for control out of the best intentions (to protect and do what is best for babies), that they can push other loving caregivers and family members away from helping them and their baby (been there, done that). These parents put themselves at risk of burnout and resentment, strain their relationship, and end up not being able to give their babies the best of themselves or what the other parent or extended family can offer, though they were so well-intentioned. Having extended family help that one can trust is a privilege that is not always available. The old adage "it takes a village" can be painful when new parents are feeling unsupported and to those parents we offer our respect for how hard you are working and compassion for how lonely you may feel.

The rates of postpartum depression and anxiety are staggering, but we want to add that those statistics only tell part of the story. In real life it is also important to acknowledge that postpartum distress is on a continuum and many, many parents struggle, even quite significantly, without meeting criteria for a diagnosis.. The stats make it seem like a subset of parents (perhaps around 25%) are struggling, while the other group is not. Yet, this is not how we see it play out. A significant proportion of the clients in our office do not have diagnoses, and we see them benefit greatly from therapy as well. We believe that understanding that postpartum distress is on a continuum can reduce stigma around it. By normalizing the struggle, new parents may feel more comfortable seeking emotional support and acknowledging the need for practical support with baby care or housework when feeling overwhelmed. It is normal to not be able to manage everything that a new baby brings particularly if one lacks outside support and this is not a failing of the parent. It really is hard.

Second, the importance of social support, in all its various forms, should not be underestimated. Parental mental health depends on it. If a new parent has a partner, the quality of that relationship strongly predicts the mental health of both partners. In our clinical practice, we work extensively on improving those relationships in terms of communication, conflict, intimacy, and on negotiating the division of labour in the home. Without specifically paying attention to the couple's relationship after baby, the relationship often takes a dive postpartum and in the early years of parenting. Taking care of the couple is taking care of the whole family.

Relationships with one's own parents is often highlighted as well after having a new baby. Practical support, emotional support, and encouragement can be crucial to a new parent's mental health. Family dynamics and unmet expectations are important topics we work with in therapy. Finally, friendships are crucial in terms of emotional sharing and staying connected with who you are as an adult, rather than solely as a parent tending to the needs of the child. While maintaining friendships from before baby is important to this end, there is also a significant benefit to making new "mommy" friends. The observation of other mothers and babies can be incredibly normalizing, especially if the others are being honest about their experiences. Whether it's a therapy or support group, baby music class, or meeting up with other parents and babies in a park, these experiences are important for a new mother getting her bearings.

We believe that fathers are lacking adequate social support even more significantly than mothers. Though many men take on a good deal of childrearing, and may even be the primary caregivers, they lack opportunities to connect with other fathers and to share openly about their experiences. We hope that this will change over time as society changes, and for now we want fathers to know that we see them struggle as well.

Third, there is no right way to parent. Let us repeat that one more time - there is no right way to parent and NO ONE has it completely figured out. Most people are trying to do their best in a difficult situation, and most of the time, it's more than good enough. Parents today face immense pressure and information overload, including conflicting advice even from well-respected sources. As a result, many parents feel they are failing. If you measure your success as a parent by how little your baby cries, by how much weight they gain, by how soundly they sleep, you are destined for a problem. Even if your baby does all these things beautifully, what happens when they don't live up to some expectation or milestone? Parents, especially mothers, often blame themselves. When a new mother looks for markers for how she is doing, she may think she is failing if she judges herself based on a newborn baby's behaviours. Babies cannot be controlled and even with a lot of effort, they still may not 'perform' the way we'd hope. We may think we are failing if baby does not gain weight at the rate we would hope, or nap according to a recommended sleep chart.

Dr. Carol Dweck, a Psychology Professor at Stanford, coined the term 'growth mindset', such that people who view difficulties as challenges yet to be overcome will be more successful at dealing with those challenges. Applying the growth mindset to new parenthood can be powerful. It means that you are still learning and growing, but that there is the possibility that you will feel more competent in the future. Try adding 'yet' to any self-doubt or self-judgement ("I don't feel like a mother... yet") or perhaps 'for now' ("I'm hating this... for now"). When Dweck describes how to build resilient kids, she advises parents to praise the process and the effort rather than the outcome (as in, "I noticed how hard you worked. That's wonderful"). Turn that to how you judge yourself. Just like Dweck would advise shifting the focus from outcome to effort for children, it follows that we would do much better noticing the effort we are putting in, and the journey itself rather than the destination. This gives us the space to become the parents we wish to be.

Fourth, parents do not need to love every minute of every stage to be a good parent. The newborn stage is often disorienting and physically demanding, toddlers are an emotional rollercoaster, and don't even get us started on teenagers! Our job as therapists isn't about helping parents to enjoy every moment but instead finding the moments that they can enjoy. People need to recognize that parenthood is a marathon, not a sprint, with many laps around the track, and their strength as a parent may be at the next lap. This does not mean that we do not try to improve mood and anxiety so that parents can be more present and joyful, but when we relax our expectations we are actually more likely to improve. Parents who have suffered from postpartum mental health challenges often express guilt about this because of the potential impact on their children. We remind them that they are seeking help, often precisely because they care so deeply for their children.

The field of perinatal mental health is hugely rewarding because we know that treatment works. We have seen first-hand the importance of support for new parents in terms of professional support and informal social support. We recognize that our practice is a private practice that is not funded by our government. We hope that in the span of our careers we will see increased access to the types of interventions that we know to be so helpful. When parents can get the help they deserve to feel better, and by extension, parent better, the benefits will be felt for generations.

Dr. Jillian Satin, a registered clinical and health psychologist, is the co-founder of The Well Parents Centre in midtown Toronto (and virtually throughout Ontario). Dr. Samantha Waxman is a registered clinical and health psychologist working with adults and couples, and is the co-founder of The Well Parents Centre. Connect with Dr. Satin and Dr. Waxman on Instagram @wellparents

WHAT ELSE COULD I DO?

Nicole Devlin

I KNEW THE MOMENT AFTER my son was born, I was experiencing something not normal. I just felt nothing. I wasn't overjoyed at the sight of him, I didn't want any visitors in the hospital to share this joy I was supposed to be feeling. I just felt blah.

This continued at home. I just felt off, not myself and not happy. I was just going through the motions of caring for this little being I had wanted so badly and was so happy to meet. I told myself, *It's just what they called the baby blues, and it would pass.* It didn't; it got worse.

With the depression came the anxiety, which I began to feel every morning. I wasn't able to eat, I was throwing up, and I couldn't take care of my son. I went to my family doctor who in turn, prescribed me medication, but my anxiety only increased. I was afraid the medication was making my anxiety worse.

A couple of days later, I found myself going to the emergency room because the anxiety was so intense. I just did not know what to do. They told me I was fine, to stop taking my medication, and to speak to my family doctor. So I went back to her, told her what had happened, that I didn't want to take the medication, and then she basically brushed me off and told me if I couldn't take what she prescribed and couldn't do what I needed to do, then she couldn't help me.

I felt defeated, lost, and once again, wound up in the hospital. This time, it was for two days with the second day landing me in the inpatient psychiatric ward. This was not a place for a new mom unsure of what was going on with her—and with no support from her family doctor. I was upset that I was just put into a room with nothing—no comforts, no explanation, and worst of all, no baby. I was alone. The doctor wanted to put me back on the same medication and continue to stay at the hospital, but I didn't want to do it because of how bad I felt the first time.

I was discharged and told to get in touch with public health and my family doctor, again. Prior to my discharge, the doctor told me that the wait time to see a psychologist was six weeks. That meant I would have to wait six full weeks with no help, but I waited. What else could I do?

When I finally did get to see the psychologist, I was surprised to see that he was a young male. I doubted he had any idea of what I was going through. I decided to go back to the family doctor's office, but this time I requested to see a different doctor.

What a difference.

This doctor listened to me while I explained everything. I was crying, and she was okay with that. Right away, she put me on a different medication to try on a low dose, and I continued to visit her once a week to slowly increase the dose. She also recommended a great psychologist. She was a private psychologist who specialized in perinatal mental health and, fortunately, I was able to afford her. I'm sad to think of moms who aren't able to afford private therapy—and why should they? Why don't we have specialized perinatal mental health therapists without long waiting lists in the areas where we need them?

She helped me figure out how I could get eating again, gave me numerous resources, and always checked in. During the darkest times, I was able to reach her on her cell after hours. She was always there to help me and calm me down. She also spoke with my husband a lot, helping us through the scary thoughts. Once I was better, she said I was one of her most severe cases of postpartum anxiety. We still keep in touch on a friendly basis, and I am forever grateful for her .

I also started attending a postpartum depression support group in town, which I had no idea existed. To know other moms out there were going through exactly what I was going through, it was life-saving to say the least.

Slowly but surely, the medication started working, the psychology visits helped, and I started to feel normal and like myself again. I am still on my medication to this day, but I know I need this to be me and the best mom I can be. I still see my doctor regularly. She has become a rock in my life. My son is now four. Although I feel I missed out on the first year with him, I truly feel a bond with him now. We are now expecting another little one and although I know the resources I can access if I were to experience postpartum depression and anxiety again, I feel that more needs to be done to help suffering moms.

This journey has turned me into a fierce perinatal mental health advocate. No mother should feel alone or stigmatized if she is going through a perinatal mental illness. I was extremely fortunate to have the support of a great family doctor and various other people in my life. My hope is that all new moms are able to access the support they need to get better.

Nicole Devlin is mom to Brady and lives in Calgary, Alberta. She is a trained peer support worker for women and families suffering with perinatal mood disorders and pregnancy loss. Connect with Nicole on Instagram @nicoledevlin

THE MYTH OF MOTHERHOOD

Jaimee Folkins

FROM THE TIME I WAS a little girl, I watched moms with their children. I imagined what it would be like to hold my baby in my arms, and all the things I would do and give to him without giving it a second thought.

Up until the day I gave birth, I had an idealized vision in my mind of what it would be like to bring a small person into the world, and the natural ways in which my life would open up easily to accommodate him.

Then, reality hit, in the form of 27 hours of hard labour, followed by an anesthetized emergency C-section, from which I was certain I would not wake up. My journey to becoming a mother was painful, terrifying, and the absolute antithesis of what I expected it to be. I had absolutely no control over my body and what was done to it, and all of the things I had planned for, had asked for, had expected, did not occur. At the end of it all, I had a beautiful baby, but I felt like I had already failed him.

As the months passed and he didn't sleep and grabbed at my skin, begging to be nursed for hours on end until I was numb and bleary eyed, I sank deeper into a well of despair. I loved my son fiercely, but every day was a struggle, and every moment felt wrapped in a thick, sticky film of anxiety and fear. When I found out that I wasn't producing enough milk, my sense that I had failed my son grew stronger and began to overshadow even the joy I felt at being his mother. *Women are made to give birth and to breastfeed*, I thought, and I couldn't even do those things right.

I watched my friends, who also had young babies and were having similar struggles to me, I felt like they were all handling it so much better. I blamed myself for the tears that sprang to my eyes far too often, and the bone deep weariness I couldn't seem to shake. I felt guilty that all I wanted more than anything in the world was to have a few hours of uninterrupted sleep, and I didn't understand how other mothers were able to leave the house and go on outings, overnight trips, and even airplanes with their babies when for me it was an accomplishment to make it to dinner time without one or both of us dissolving into uncontrollable sobs.

I listened to other women tell their birth stories, using descriptors like *amazing, magical,* and *powerful,* and I felt a deep sense of shame that every time I thought of the day my son came into the world I felt like my throat was closing over and I couldn't breathe. For the first six months, when strangers and friends would ask me how I was enjoying motherhood, I wanted to scream at them (and sometimes I did), that it was nothing like I thought, and that even though I had been doing it for such a short time, what I really needed more than anything was a break.

I was offered help, and sometimes I took it, but most of the time, despite the fact that I felt like I was drowning in the days and weeks, I wanted to wrap myself and my son in a bubble, hidden from the world, where no one else could touch us. The Internet was my best friend and my worst enemy, as I pored over websites telling me all the things I could do better, and all the things I'd already done that were certain to scar my son for life. I knew that how I was feeling wasn't normal, wasn't healthy, and wasn't okay, but I wasn't sure how to ask for help for myself, when my world had shifted to center around this new little human I had created.

Six months after my son was born, I dug deep within myself and sought out counselling, pouring out my feelings of inadequacy and my overwhelming, all-encompassing love for my son to a woman who proceeded to tell me that I was *unhealthily enmeshed* with the baby, and that unless I loosened my grip, he was sure to end up living in my basement forever. I promptly stopped seeing her and once again kept my thoughts and feelings to myself.

When my son was 11 months old, I went back to work and felt a little bit of my old self creeping back. I realized I had missed work, and with this realization came the crushing guilt that I hadn't in fact *enjoyed every moment* of being home with my son the way all the well-meaning women whose children were old enough that they'd forgotten the particular hell that was sleep deprivation had insisted I should.

Then, when my son was 13 and a half months old, I went to Las Vegas for six days for a conference, never having left him before that for more than a few hours at a time, and we were both okay. Around that same time, he started sleeping through the night, and the hours of unbroken rest and time to myself healed me in ways nothing else could have. I also started therapy, giving myself permission to try to tell my story one more time, revealing myself in all my perceived flaws and hoping that the mirror that was held up to reflect them wasn't too sharp and unforgiving.

This counsellor, a strong, smart, compassionate woman, gave me back yet another piece of myself when she told me how strong she thought I was for having survived such a difficult year. She also told me that she thought I might be suffering from postpartum anxiety, and also features of postpartum post-traumatic stress disorder. In that moment, something clicked. A large part of me wanted to reject that particular terminology, because I felt like claiming it as my own would somehow take away from the trauma suffered by veterans, police officers, paramedics, and survivors of abuse. My counsellor helped me see that my experience was just as valid as other people's, and that my road to healing couldn't begin until I let myself believe that I was just as worthy of care and support as anyone else.

From the time we are little girls, many of us dream of becoming mothers. We hold our dolls close and sing to them, maneuver their stiff arms and legs into different outfits, and tuck them in at night. We learn early on that love, when you're female, means giving, means nurturing, means taking care of others and putting their needs before our own. We learn that asking for too much for ourselves makes us needy, makes us selfish, and that speaking up too loudly or too often, asking for the things we want makes us bossy, bitchy, shrewish, and more than a little bit unlovable.

Standing here, on the other side of a year in which all of my notions of what it means to be a woman and a mother were challenged, I feel as though I finally understand that it's okay to take as much as you give, and that asking for what you need looks a hell of a lot more like strength than it does weakness.

As my counsellor helped me find my way back to myself and I watched my baby continue to grow and thrive, still as connected to me as he was separate, I found myself wondering why it had taken more than a year for anyone to acknowledge that my racing thoughts, my all-consuming fear, and the flashbacks that constricted my chest and stole my breath weren't a *normal* part of the experience of being a new mother; why no one had listened more closely or asked any follow-up questions when I had told them (and I had told them, more than once) that I wasn't okay.

I began to talk to other women, other mothers, who felt lost and sad and afraid, and I began to realize not only that I wasn't alone, but that I wasn't inexcusably flawed, and I wasn't failing my son. I was anxious, and I had been traumatized by a birth experience that was out of my control, during which I had felt my life was at risk, and this had necessarily altered my perception of the world. I also realized that, with help, I could feel better. This glimmer of hope that was offered to me by my counsellor made me want to offer the same thing to other mothers. I was a counselling therapist already, with thoughts of pursuing a career as a school counsellor once my maternity leave had ended, but I began to think about how I could help other mothers instead. I decided to take additional training through Postpartum Support International to specialize in perinatal mental health.

The baby boy who pushed and shaped and grew and stretched me past the lengths of who I thought I was and into who I now know myself to be will turn six years old soon. My whole world still fits inside his smile, and his little sister's, too. Parenthood is a paradox: You're never alone and yet it can be so lonely. One of the greatest gifts we can give each other as mothers is to tell the truth of our experience, in all its heartache and joy, so that we can see ourselves reflected in one another, and together we can heal.

Jaime Folkins is a mom of two and lives in Fredericton, New Brunswick. She owns a counselling practice called Balanced Beginnings Counselling Therapy (can be found on Facebook) and works primarily with women in all stages of their parenting journey, from conception to parenting and beyond, including pregnancy loss and infertility. You can find Jaimee on Instagram @abalancedbeginning

SUFFOCATING STEREOTYPES

Rosa Caporicci

THE SCENE IS SEARED INTO my memory. Me, standing at the kitchen counter, looking at a bunch of cleaned baby bottles, convinced that this would never end. By that point, I had forced myself to give up the battle that I would somehow learn to love breastfeeding, and had burned through countless brands of regular formula, soy formula, anything that would help my daughter eat without the ubiquitous bouts of projectile vomiting, just something that would quiet her ceaseless crying. Nothing seemed to help.

Her birth had been a godsend after my experience delivering her sister. That event was an 18-hour marathon, culminating with two nurses pushing on my abdomen while my doctor applied the ventose, which resulted in a third-degree tear even with the episiotomy she had performed. I remember believing I would never walk again.

This time, I remember talking to myself not to panic when I learned that the anaesthesiologist could not be called back to administer an epidural. Although I literally thought the waves of pain radiating down my thighs were strong enough to crack my bones, I was relieved that her arrival three hours later resulted in no tearing.

My daughter in those first few adrenaline-soaked heady days was sedate and calm, as all newborns seem to be. However, it wasn't long before what is colloquially called colic set in and my world turned upside down. Worry turned into frustration, which turned into rage, which turned into desperation and hopelessness.

While I had struggled with mood problems for the better part of my life—initially with anxiety as a kid, then descending into depression following the death of my father when I was twelve—I had blithely either ignored or plowed through difficult periods. This included what was quite likely a postpartum mood and anxiety disorder after having my first child, highlighted by my initial confrontation with the shocking discovery that I was not enamoured with breastfeeding despite my assumptions reinforced by the clarion call of *breast is best!* This, however, was altogether different.

I remember my family doctor remarking that I wasn't my usual chipper self when I saw her for my six-week wellness check. I was listless and wrung out not only from the demands of a high-needs baby, but from my own constant crying. Days earlier, I had punched a hole in the basement wall, the pent-up energy of wanting to escape, having nowhere else to go. And I count myself lucky. I've always joked that my husband has the patience of Job; without his support, both material and emotional, I don't know how much further I would have fallen.

That walk home from the pharmacy with my prescription for an antidepressant in hand cemented for me my worst fear. *I'm officially crazy*, I thought. Within weeks, though, the fog of depression began to lift, and I had a renewed sense of myself; so much so, that I reinitiated my job search (having been fired during my pregnancy because I was pregnant. Fear not, it resulted in a settlement). I landed a job, which kickstarted the beginning of a long road to a career reorientation, and decided that I was a better mother working than being at home, even before my maternity leave expired. My husband and I were happy to exchange jobs.

Fast forward ten years and that long career path found me back in graduate school. When I earned my M.A. in Counselling Psychology, I had not intended to work in private practice, nor did I have any idea that I would ultimately specialize in maternal mental health. The idea came to me over time when I realized that while the medication I had taken was instrumental in treating my symptoms, I wasn't given any psychosocial support, either during my postpartum period or following the death of our son whom I laboured and delivered almost a year to the day before his sister was born.

I set my mind to learning about and training in reproductive mental health, and to use my skills as a psychotherapist to ensure as best I could that no other mother, parent, or family would suffer needlessly.

Almost ten years later, I have met and treated over 500 clients and families, and I've learned a few things. Chief among them is that the assumption that childbearing and childrearing is the zenith of a woman's life continues to be as deeply entrenched in our society as it is insidious. The danger with this belief is that it not only cuts women and families off from finding support (how can you ask for help when you're convinced you're not supposed to be unhappy?), it literally cuts women off from themselves. Add to that the suffocating stereotypes of intensive mothering promulgated by social media and it's no wonder the prevalence of perinatal mood and anxiety disorders is so high.

As I have grown accustomed to telling my clients, you were a person before becoming pregnant and having a baby; she hasn't gone anywhere, nor should she. It is wholly unhealthy to accept the societal expectation that a woman should be content in having her personhood subsumed by motherhood, but that's what I find so many of my clients striving to do. I have even grown allergic to the idea that motherhood is a role. I consider it anathema. If we looked at motherhood as a job—as work—which in my view it is, we could then examine the structural elements that I believe contribute to the high rates of maternal mood disorders.

What job do you know requires you to work 24 hours a day, seven days a week, with no remuneration, breaks, or vacation time? Is it not possible that social policies (like maternity leaves, read: women), which favour the mother almost exclusively, leave her to almost single-handedly care for an infant, reinforces the idea that this is normal and what she should want to do? Is it not conceivable that so-called baby friendly, but mother-hurtful hospital initiatives, which place the ideologies of breastfeeding ahead of a woman's mental health needs are detrimental to her well-being? Is an industry that places natural childbirth on a pedestal and at any cost profoundly misogynistic when it ignores the emotional, physical, and mental costs to women?

As I often also say to my clients, we make a fundamental error when we conflate the love we have for our children with the lack of or absence of appreciation we may have for the job of childrearing. The fact that women may acknowledge the drudgery, monotony and bone-crushing work of taking care of a vulnerable human being does not mean they don't love their baby; they are separate and distinct. Two things can be true at the same time. We then, collaboratively, take the time to re-learn how to reconnect with her desires and needs, a disconnection that should have never happened in the first place.

So, while I may have long recovered from the that which was depression and anxiety for which the perinatal experience was a catalyst, I am also cognizant of how my passion to help women and families was borne from that experience. I hope the work I am privileged to do with women helps them re-discover their innate strengths and assets to become the best parent they can be for their child and their family, which is as it should be, as unique as they are, and which hopefully frees them from the tyranny of what it is to be a good mother.

Rosa Caporicci is a licensed psychotherapist in private practice (NDG Therapy) and lives in Montreal with her high school teacher-husband and three late-teen, young adult daughters (plus Hudson, the rescue dog and his somewhat tolerant feline buddies, Tigger and Nemo). She is the Quebec coordinator for Postpartum Support International and is a member of PLIDA (Pregnancy Loss & Infant Death Alliance), CFAS (Canadian Fertility & Andrology Society), MONA (Marcé Society of North America) and Fertility Matters Canada. You can learn more about her practice at https://www.ndgtherapy.com, as well as matters that interest her and her clientele through her Facebook page at https://www.facebook.com/ndgtherapy/.

YOU'RE NOT MEANT TO DO THIS ALONE

Sheila Duffy

I SUFFERED FROM SEVERE DEPRESSION and anxiety during my pregnancy and postpartum with my first child. At that time, almost 30 years ago, there was very little information about postpartum mood disorders and although I had most of the risk factors, there was no screening for perinatal mental illness or monitoring from my doctor or even discussion around the fact that I was high risk.

During my pregnancy, I began to have terrible intrusive thoughts. The thoughts were upsetting and confusing, and I did not understand what was happening. I was worried that the thoughts I was having were premonitions that I would harm my baby. Not only was I afraid of the thoughts, I was terrified that I might act on them. I had no idea how to get help. I began to heavily doubt myself and thought that this meant I wasn't equipped to be a mother and that it was somehow about my personal inadequacies rather than perinatal anxiety, which is a condition that affects one in five women. If I had that information then, it may have made a difference in the outcome and manageability of my emotions. I certainly would have sought help sooner.

I had a very difficult and traumatic birth experience, which I also believe contributed and snowballed into more issues postpartum. I had difficulties with breastfeeding, a high-needs baby, all of which I attributed to mean that I was not supposed to be a mom. I felt I was failing at all of it. Everything pointed back to me being the problem. My baby cried a lot and was hard to soothe, and I blamed myself. My husband worked long hours and neither of our families lived nearby, so I was left on my own for very long days with no support. This led to extreme stress for my partner and I. We were both sleep deprived and exhausted and constantly pushed beyond our capacity. We were completely unprepared for the stress we were experiencing with the adjustment to parenthood. This caused intense marital strain, and we were both angry at each other. I felt that he did not understand and that his expectations were unrealistic of me. He felt stretched at work and at home, unable to meet the expectations anywhere. We both felt a lot of blame and that the other person was part of the problem.

I think I would have gotten better sooner if I had treatment and support. But without understanding anything about perinatal mental illness, I suffered for a long time. Eventually, I did start to feel better as my baby got older and around the one-year mark, it was easier and felt more manageable. I finally began to enjoy my baby and motherhood. Not long after that, I found out I was pregnant again, and the symptoms returned. Anxiety and intrusive thoughts that I was going to harm my baby resurfaced and now with the second baby on the way, things were much more complicated, partly because of the fact that I had not had treatment or support with my first.

My postpartum experience was much worse with the second baby. I had extreme anxiety and suicidal thinking. Things escalated quickly and at my worst, I contemplated suicide as not only a solution to my despair, but that my family would be better off without me.

It was a long road to recovery. Just like there were a lot of contributing factors to my postpartum experience, there were also lots of things that helped me to get better. What was different the second time around was that I had support, which made a huge difference. It took some time for me to get well, but this time, I was not suffering alone. I had people who understood, and I received compassionate non-judgmental support though the Pacific Post Partum Society support group.

Getting support not only saved my life, it also changed my life in a profound way. I began to get more practical help and much needed breaks. I started to understand that it was not a weakness on my part to need breaks and to need help. The more attention I paid to my needs and the more I acknowledged and respected my limitations, the better I felt. I started to see myself as unique. I had my own unique way of being a mother so rather than trying to fit myself into the version of motherhood and unrealistic myths and expectations of what it meant to be a mother, I started to question and challenge those expectations. I realized that in some ways, we are set up to fail and that we are not meant to do this job on our own. Yet many of us are. We were meant to do this with a village of support, and it was less about me not being good enough and more about societal issues like lack of support and unrealistic expectations that were contributing to my sense of failure. I started to understand what my needs were and that they were vitally important as I was the emotional center of our family. If I was not okay, no one was okay. My needs were important, and my children seeing that my needs were important was also good for them.

Although I would not wish this experience on anyone, I am grateful today that I did go through this as the things I truly value in my life came from this dark time. Today, I am surrounded by a community of support as a result of this experience. I no longer suffer through anything alone and I have a deep understanding of self-care and how all of us do not need to travel through difficult transitions in life without support. I found the Pacific Post Partum Support Society when my son was three weeks old and I've basically never left. I became involved with PPPSS after my experience and I have had the incredible privilege of working with postpartum moms for the last 25 years. I have heard many stories. I sit with women who share their scariest thoughts and feelings, and I witness their courageous journeys of recovery from a dark and difficult time. I watch them come through to the other side and listen to them as they share their success and gifts they have received as a result...just as I did.

Sheila Duffy is a mom of two and lives in Vancouver, British Columbia. She is the Director of the Pacific Post Partum Support Society and has been providing telephone support, group facilitation, and counselling for over 25 years. You can connect with Sheila on Instagram @sheilahaldane and @pacificpostpartum

•

MINDFULNESS

Laurel Hicks

I BECAME INTERESTED IN PERINATAL mental health in a very accidental way, through yoga.

Yoga is my passion. I love it so much that I became a yoga teacher. I spent my days as an engineer and my nights teaching yoga.

I was happy but felt something was missing.

Then my sister became pregnant and wanted to practice prenatal yoga but she couldn't take any classes or advice from me because I didn't have any formal training in prenatal yoga. When I looked into it more I began to really enjoy learning about how to take care of a moms-to-be during pregnancy and beyond.

Though I didn't have any children of my own, I could feel myself becoming more and more passionate about perinatal health and perinatal mental health in particular.

Twelve beautiful expecting women showed up to my very first prenatal yoga class and I was hooked. I began learning from them how stressed some women were in pregnancy, and how much they craved community.

I also realized how much I didn't know about this time of life. This pretty much set me on a path to gain more knowledge about perinatal mental health. I became a labour doula and then as a masters of social work student.

Bye-bye engineering, hello moms and babies!

I became so enthralled about perinatal mental health and making a difference that I trained as a therapist, which eventually led me to pursue a dual-title PhD in social work and infant mental health. Now my research focuses on ways to improve wellness and resilience in families during the prenatal and postnatal period. My research specifically focuses on trauma-informed and mindfulness-based practices.

I am currently researching the effects of an online-mindfulness intervention to prevent relapse of depression in pregnant people.

We know that past episodes of depression is a huge risk factor for relapse of depression during pregnancy and postpartum. The study I'm working on, funded by the NIMH (led by Principal investigators Sona Dimidjian, PhD and Lee Cohen, MD) focuses on teaching skills while people are feeling emotionally well that may help them to reduce their risk of depression relapse.

The program that we are teaching the women is a technology-delivered mindfulness-based cognitive therapy (MBCT) program that is specifically designed for pregnant and postpartum women.

It is an eight-session online (asynchronous) program called Mindful Mood Balance for Moms. The program has been delivered in person and a small pilot was delivered through this online program.

The research so far has shown that it is effective in reducing relapse of depression. This is so important because if we can keep people well in pregnancy and postpartum, this not only affects the pregnant person's wellbeing but also their entire family system, including their infant's behavior and development.

This study in particular is the brainchild of Sona Dimidjian, PhD and Zindel Segal, PhD. I am interested in this work because I see the benefits of teaching MBCT and yoga with pregnant women and I am incredibly passionate about improving wellness during pregnancy and postpartum.

I love the idea of prevention as well. So much of our mental health system is focused on responding to a crisis instead of employing ways to prevent them. By focusing on improving wellness in pregnancy, it will hopefully be the ultimate prevention by improving the wellness of the infant starting in utero.

Dr. Hicks received a dual-title Ph.D. in social work (clinical concentration) and infant mental health from Wayne State University. She is also a licensed clinical social worker and a certified perinatal mental health therapist (PMH-C) and has a private practice in Denver, CO. She is licensed in Colorado and Michigan and can offer online therapy in both locations. She is trained in interpersonal therapy, mindfulness-based cognitive therapy, EMDR, CBT, trauma-informed yoga therapy and integrates mind-body approaches into treatment with her clients. She also offers prenatal yoga, prenatal yoga teacher trainings and mindfulness-based stress reduction classes. Connect with Laurel on Instagram @mindfulmamasyoga

A GOOD FRIEND

Dr. Phillippa Houghton

POSTPARTUM AND NEW MOTHERHOOD ARE hard, much harder than pregnancy, labour, and birth—and yet what do all the classes prepare you for? Certainly not the emotional journey you will walk as you navigate one of the biggest transitions of your life—becoming a mother.

I thought somehow, my years of medical training would prepare me for this moment. I knew about birth, I knew about physical recovery, I (thought) I knew about newborns. I felt prepared—but I (like many women) was gobsmacked by all the things I was NOT prepared for, all the things I wish someone had warned me about.

I was not prepared for the newborn sleep patterns, the real physical recovery, the breastfeeding struggles, the cluster feeding, the dichotomy of never having a moment to myself whilst also feeling the weight of loneliness that comes with being home full time with a newborn. It caught me off guard.

The fact that I felt so under prepared for this transition, as a family medicine resident; someone who theoretically specializes in families, got me thinking that most women must also feel equally unsteady in their new roles. Most women must feel uncertain, out of control, and out of sorts—at least to a certain extent, no matter what their circumstances or background experience.

Full disclosure, I have not walked the journey of perinatal mood or anxiety disorders personally; but I am passionate about this topic because someone close to me has. While it took me a few weeks to find my footing in new motherhood, with the support and love of some experienced mama friends and family, I started to feel confident in my new role. I have never forgotten that wobbly feeling of the early days, and I am keenly aware of how a few vulnerabilities can quickly turn a short-term wobble into a full-blown illness.

Dr. Alexandra Sacks said, "When a baby is born, so is a mother, each unsteady in their own way" and it is this unsteady feeling that comes with newborn motherhood that has inspired me to open my heart to this population.

When I was close to a year postpartum, a good friend reached out to me for help. She was a new mama, a few weeks in, and she was scared. She was scared because she didn't feel like herself. She felt anxious. She was tearful. She wasn't sleeping. At all. She had lost her joy, her spark, her appetite, her confidence, and her purpose. She felt she was failing her infant, that her baby deserved better. She was terrified of making a mistake, hypervigilant to everything, feeding volumes, diaper changes, sleep patterns. Everything. She was suffering.

My heart went out to her, and I wanted to do everything I could to support her. However, I was suddenly conscious of my lack of knowledge and experience in the topic of perinatal mental health. I knew the basics of course but not enough. So, I learned alongside her. As I supported her through her journey, I did my own research with the intention that should any of my patients ever be in similar circumstances I would be prepared to give them the best care possible.

Since that time, I am so proud to share that, with appropriate treatment, my friend has recovered and is thriving as a mama. Her story has pushed me to pursue certification in perinatal mental health and to focus a portion of my practice on the management of these conditions at the primary care level. It dawned on me that, given most episodes of perinatal mental illness do fall into the mild-moderate range, we as family doctors have so much potential and power to identify, support, and manage these women and their families early. The faster an unwell mama is identified and treated, the faster we can get her back on track to enjoying her transition to motherhood.

Every mama deserves a happy and healthy perinatal experience, and every baby deserves a happy and healthy mama. Don't be afraid to come forward, it is not your fault and with help you will be well again.

Dr. Phillippa Houghton decided to pursue training through Postpartum Support International and is passionate about sharing her knowledge to reduce stigma around perinatal mental health. She can be found on social media at @makingmamawell and www.makingmamawell.ca

A WORD FOR THE DADS

Mark Williams

MY WIFE, MICHELLE, HAD TO have an emergency C-section for the birth of our son. It was a traumatic experience, and I was scared. I thought she was going to die. Thankfully, both Michelle and our new baby boy, Ethan, were okay. But what became apparent soon after was that Michelle began suffering from postpartum anxiety and depression.

I remember at the time having dreams about how both my loved ones had died during the procedure and having vivid thoughts about the knives on the table next to me. I would wake up thinking it was all real, but little did I know just how real things would get when Michelle went on to have severe postnatal depression. My wonderful wife, Michelle, totally changed, and it was horrible watching your loved one going through this daily. I would have given up everything, any amount of money, for her to be well.

I was so uneducated about mental health that I'd think, *How can people be depressed? How does that happen?* Within weeks, I had to leave my job to care for Michelle and Ethan.

I'd loved the social side of my work, and now I was totally isolated; I didn't even get out the front door for days. My personality quickly changed, and I started drinking more to cope. I became angry to the point that when I did manage to get out with friends, I wanted to fight the doorman to get hurt and stop these thoughts I was getting in my head. I even broke my hand after punching the sofa when Ethan was about six months. This was totally out of character for me. I began having suicidal thoughts and could not control them.

I knew I had to be strong and look after my wife and my baby. But the truth is, I was not well either. I struggled on without telling anyone. I was afraid of people knowing and it going on medical records if I changed careers. I did not know anyone who had suffered from postpartum depression, certainly not any dads so I kept up my smiley appearance and kept going. I did not want it to affect Michelle's mental health.

There were days I would draw the curtains and did not want to talk to people, which was a first for me.

The problem was that, at the time, I did not feel like I could talk to anyone. I was brought up in a working-class community where my father and his father were coal miners. I had to *man up* in my way of thinking. As much as we are a close family, there was not much emotion shown when things were tough, and I always kept it suppressed inside like a gas bottle ready to explode.

Michelle's postpartum depression lasted around 18 months, and the not knowing how long she would be unwell for was the hardest part. And of course it affected our relationship, which might well have ended as happens to so many families with no early prevention during this time. I started lying to Michelle. I would tell her I was going to work, but in fact I was isolating myself from people. I did not see the point of it all at times and felt totally alone.

I suffered mood changes for years. Then my grandfather died and within a few weeks, my beloved mother was diagnosed with cancer. She later recovered, but I thought I was going to lose her as well. My symptoms intensified. I was experiencing intrusive thoughts and nightmares, and one day had a complete breakdown in my car before work.

Eventually, I was put on medication, took a course of cognitive behavioural therapy and mindfulness, and I was lucky to be able to turn things around. I was so glad to be offered the help and engaged in everything I could. I was later diagnosed with attention deficit hyperactivity disorder, which I had managed without knowing for years. I know now that I suffered from postpartum depression too.

But I was never diagnosed with paternal postpartum depression or post-traumatic stress disorder as there was no screening for me and I was never asked about my own mental health. I was lucky I survived but that isn't the case for many new fathers and the relationships sadly end due to lack of communication and understanding that any new parents can struggle as we know the lack of sleep on its own can impact on our mental health.

Fatherhood is the best job in the world ,and I have now changed my life for the better. I am now an advocate for paternal postpartum depression, and I share my story as much as I can.

Fatherhood has changed in recent years. There are many more single dads and stay-at-home fathers than ever before. Fathers are now more actively involved in their children's day to day lives.

For many, the transition to fatherhood is a very joyful experience. Hhowever for some, it can also be a very stressful time that can trigger mental health issues.

What is really alarming is that many fathers are more at risk of suicide during the perinatal period than at any other time in their life (Quevedo 2011). If fathers are not supported at this important time, it can have a massive impact on the whole family and on the development of the child.

Antenatal perinatal mental health education for dads is the way forward. Fathers need to be educated about how their mental health can be affected by becoming a dad and what they can do to get help and support for themselves and their family. Fathers also need to be educated about the signs to look out for which indicate that their partner may have perinatal mental health concerns. Supporting both moms and dads at this critical time is essential.

Some fathers have a past history of trauma, anxiety, and depression before they become a parent. The lack of sleep associated with looking after a newborn and the transition into fatherhood can cause anxiety and depression too.

Movember in 2019 reported that one in five British fathers felt totally isolated during their first year of fatherhood. The National Childbirth Trust UK said in 2015 that 38 percent of dads had struggled with their mental health and 73 percent were worried about their partner's mental health. Fathers witnessing a traumatic birth can suffer from post traumatic stress disorder, an anxiety disorder that is brought on by either witnessing or experiencing a life-threatening event.

If you're a dad, don't suffer in silence. Speak to someone today.

Mark Williams is the author of *Daddy Blues: Postnatal Depression and Fatherhood*, and the founder of International Fathers Mental Health Day and the #HowAreYouDad campaign. He is an avid international advocate for paternal mental health and lives in the U.K. with his wife and Ethan, their son.

Part 3:

Postpartum Anger

WELL, I'M NOT

"How are you feeling, love?" they say.
But, I don't know how to reply.
There's a liquid fear sliding down my throat
And I'm being suffocated inside.

"How are you coping, love?", they ask.
When I know I'm obviously not.
Why's there an assumption that I must cope?
I'm learning to deal with an awful lot.

I haven't had a full night's sleep,
My mind has turned to mush.
I feel I'm always on high alert.
This mum thing's really tough.

"How can I help you, love?", they say.
Just pop over for a friendly chat.
Let me feel like I'm not alone in this;
It's overwhelming from where I'm sat.

"What do you need, love?", they ask.
Take the reins for just one morning.
Let me not cope 'til I've figured it out,
Without making me feel like I'm not coping.

Leander Moore
@postpartumpoet

INTERNAL FURY

Talia Singer

I WAS A NURSE, SO of course, after seeing many patients with perinatal mental health issues I didn't recognize the same symptoms in myself. I never expected to feel this way. I did not allow myself to admit that I had postpartum depression, and the shame of it was beyond bearable.

I was 27 when my first child was born and I had what they refer to as an uneventful pregnancy, but for me, it felt quite magical. Each day, each week, I allowed myself to read about every eyelash and toenail in development, a miniature magical world growing inside me. What I failed to realize was that I had spent exactly 40 weeks preparing to be pregnant, but nothing could prepare me for the experience of motherhood.

At 38 weeks, 12 hours of labor, Pitocin, and a few pushes, her little head and arms were halfway out. My doctor instructed me to reach down and pull her out myself the rest of the way. I hesitated for a second, and half-terrified she would be trapped between worlds, I reached down and pulled my 8 pound, 4 ounce daughter onto my chest. She was a perfect, chubby-cheeked cherub and as I gazed down at her, I knew instantaneously that I felt absolutely nothing.

By nothing, I mean I was devoid of feeling. I was numb. I knew it as I lay looking at her, appreciating her the way one might appreciate a sculpture at the Musée Rodin, but when I touched her, it was me that felt cold on her silky warm skin. I didn't want to say anything to anyone, even though the dark thoughts were there so soon after her birth. I told myself I was in shock, that it was the effects of the epidural, or that I was sleep deprived. We packed up from the hospital and went home 48 hours after her birth, and I placed her in her crib in her room, stared at her, and waited for some emotion to fill me.

Eventually, after a few days, an emotion did find me, and it was anger. The anger, which began as small frustrations, became an internal fury. Every time I couldn't get her to latch properly, I felt like I wanted to jump out of an eighth story window of our condo. I wanted to hit my husband. I wanted to throw myself against sharp objects. I wanted to smash all the plates in the kitchen.

When I did sleep, which was in fitful 60-minute intervals, I only dreamed of death, and blood, and blue, cold babies. People would call the house to ask how I was doing, and I mostly lied.

One time, my parents called and I told my mother the truth, that I had been staring at the balcony and trying to think of reasons not to jump off. Upon hearing this, she asked if she could take me to the hospital and I angrily hung up on her. My dreams then started to include visions of me on a psychiatric unit with my daughter apprehended by child services. I started to keep everything to myself.

My first visit to the family doctor, about six weeks postpartum, had my doctor going through a checklist placed on a clipboard. She was engrossed in her questions and did not make any eye contact. As she moved down the list of standard postnatal questions, she got to, *any depression?*

"Yes," I responded.

"Any support at home?" she asked

"Yes" I responded again.

It was true. I did have support at home if I needed it. My husband came home in the evenings and helped. If I needed my family, they would be there for me. I just couldn't let anyone know what I was really thinking. My doctor's eyes never left the page when I responded yes to feelings of depression, she did not ask me to elaborate, and she never followed up. I often wonder if she had, would I have told her that each day at 8 a.m., when my husband left the house, my routine consisted of me thinking of reasons not to die?

I got into a kind of routine where I just accepted the thoughts of death accompanying me everywhere I went with my baby. If we were driving on the highway to get to a mommy and me class, the thoughts of crashing into oncoming traffic rode alongside me in the passenger seat. If I took her for a walk in the stroller in the park, the thought of me abandoning the stroller walked along beside me, and when I put her to bed in her crib, I tucked her in with the thought that she might not wake up.

My daughter grew bigger, and cooed and walked, and ate solid foods, and went to baby classes, and did this despite the fact that I was smiling on the outside and completely desolate on the inside. I felt like one of those haunted mansions that look like they could be charming on the outside but are charred internally from a terrible fire. When the anger subsided, I felt that all of my anatomy consisted of carbonised bones and organs made of coal.

I lived like this for about three years. And then I found psychoanalysis, a type of therapy that helped me express my darkest thoughts. I felt accepted by my therapist. He understood how I felt. *How strange*, I thought, *for a man to know what it was like for me, a mother, to look at my daughter and feel nothing*. He showed me a new level of compassion I had never received before. I spent nearly ten years in analysis and found myself again. I cannot express the ways in which this therapy helped me to be a better mother, have an emotionally loving relationship with my first and then second born, and help me shed the shame of postpartum depression. I still remember it sometimes, the guilt. The depression which was masked in anger was short lived, but the guilt of it nearly killed me.

Talia Singer is a mom of two and lives in Toronto, Ontario. She is a registered nurse and psychotherapist as well as the host of a podcast about psychotherapy called WhateverWorks. You can find Talia on Instagram @whateverworkspod and at https://www.taliasinger.com/whateverworks-podcast/

BLINDING RAGE

Susan Sinclair

THINGS YOU EXPECT TO FEEL in the weeks after having your first child: joy, love, exhaustion, confusion, apprehension, anxiety, and even weepiness. Things you don't expect to feel in the weeks after having your first child: blinding RAGE.

I was angry at everything, angry that the baby was crying, angry at my husband for anything that did. In the blink of an eye, I could go from the most loving, caring mom, to feeling the most intense anger I'd ever felt. And after the rage, came the guilt. *How can I think that way about my beautiful new baby?* I started to isolate myself, not wanting to talk to anyone, fearing that if I were to say out loud the things I was thinking, any sane person would call child services and my baby would most certainly be taken away from me.

I was flying into rages for over two months before my family doctor noticed that I seemed off. During a routine appointment with my then three-and-a-half-month-old son, she asked me how I was coping.

"Not great," I replied.

She talked about postpartum depression.

"Do you think you may have it?" she asked me.

"No!" I exclaimed "I'm not sad at all."

"Let's talk about it a bit more," she said to me kindly.

She started listing the other symptoms of perinatal mental illness, the ones you never hear about. When she got to anger, I immediately sat up and acknowledged to her that yes, I was having major fits of rage, quite frequently actually. I was prescribed a low dose of an antidepressant, and was reassured that it was completely safe for nursing mothers.

Then I talked to my husband. That was harder than talking to my doctor. My husband admitted that he absolutely knew that something was wron, but had been afraid to say anything because of how I had been reacting to simple everyday things (I once threw a box of diapers at him!). He was worried that I would fly off the handle if he were to bring it up. I think that was the worst part, realizing how my perinatal mental illness was affecting his ability to communicate with me.

The antidepressant was able to provide me with a few more inches of fuse before I blew up, but that's all it did. It didn't stop the intrusive thoughts I started having about my son and me. I still have guilt from these thoughts to this day. I had frequent thoughts about getting in my car and driving away and never coming back. I also had thoughts of driving head on into a transport truck.

I didn't talk about these thoughts. I didn't dare tell anyone about these thoughts. I couldn't tell anyone because I really and truly believed that my son would be taken away from me.

For seven months, I suffered in silence. For seven months, I pretended that everything was great while being completely tortured with these horrible, intrusive thoughts.

Then I broke. Seven weeks before I was scheduled to go back to work, I got called into my office and was told I was being terminated, that they had restructured and there was no place for me. Fortunately, I had a law degree and knew my rights, so I called a lawyer within hours.

That event completely broke me and prompted me to tell my husband and my doctor about my intrusive thoughts. Within a week, I was in individual and group therapy, both specific to dealing with women dealing with perinatal mental illness.

Therapy was a game-changer for me. No one took my son away. No one shamed me or made me feel guilty for the thoughts I had been having. In group therapy, I discovered that perinatal mental illness can affect any woman of any status, race, or age. A lot of the women in the support group had the same intrusive thoughts I had been having. I finally learned that I wasn't alone. I wasn't crazy, and I wasn't a bad mom. If anything, I learned that I was actually a great mom; a great mom who was finally able to recognize that she was sick and needed some help in order to provide the best care for her child.

That was the biggest eye-opener for me, realizing that a mental illness is the same as a physical illness. You wouldn't not take insulin if you were diagnosed with diabetes. Medication and therapy were my treatment, and that treatment was necessary for me to survive.

Being a mom means doing hard things, and sometimes the hardest thing is to ask for the help you need. Taking that first step of asking for help and actually saying out loud the way I was feeling was, without a doubt, the hardest part of the process. And now, I openly talk about it. I talk about it with people the same way I would talk about a physical illness. I want society to move away from not talking about mental illness, to stop treating it like a dirty little taboo secret. I think perinatal mental illness is one of the least talked about mental illnesses, because of the societal expectations that are put upon mothers. The shame and stigma must stop and we need to talk about it, especially the rage that makes us so afraid.

To the other moms struggling with a perinatal mental illness, please know, you are not alone. You are not a bad mom. You deserve help, medical care, and experienced mental health services. You deserve to feel better for you, and your family. You are worth it, and it will get better.

Susan Sinclair is a mom of two and lives in Guelph, Ontario. She is a plant loving, crystal collecting, grey-haired, tattooed, Aquarian empath, who also manages to enjoy a successful career in corporate human resources. She can be found on Instagram @not.your.averagemama where she talks about motherhood, mental health, and menopause.

ELLA BELLA

Elita Paterson

GIVING BIRTH WAS MY LIFE'S worst fear. I think that's why I may have waited so long to have a baby. It all started when my dad showed me at age six, on TV, how a baby was really born. Nope, the baby did not come out of your belly button, as I was told on several occasions. The baby comes out of where you pee from!

I. WAS. HORRIFIED.

Although, I'm not sure how less painful it would be if the baby came out of my belly button?!

Even after this traumatic experience, I still wanted a baby a couple decades later. Sadly, after a painful miscarriage, I felt an extreme sense of failure instead of grief. I went through a mild depression. I started taking lots of sick days from work and closing all the curtains in our house. I just wanted to be alone.

Five months later, I was overjoyed to be pregnant again. Our Ella Bella was born March 13th, 2006 at 3:30 a.m. and I'm thrilled to say that my birthing experience was so positive. The nurses were amazing and even a midwife got to deliver our Ella Bella as she came earlier than the doctor anticipated. I was thrilled for all the support and that the epidural worked.

My husband, Ward, and I were thrilled, but our new baby Ella? Not so much. She cried for nearly an hour afterward because she had meconium extracted out of her nose and mouth before given to us. It was like she was born with the pedal to the metal being so revved-up all the time.

There was no comforting her, and breastfeeding didn't come easy either. I began to feel extremely incompetent, anxious, scared, and angry. The anger turned into fits of rage as the months passed where I couldn't comfort Ella well at all. I would get so close to shaking her, and would push her down hard on the couch or bed or crib while being swaddled-up tightly, instead, while yelling, "What the hell do I do, now? HELP ME!"

After my rages and realizing how I could have really hurt Ella, I became excessively guilt-ridden and shameful. I just wish I realized at that time, I simply didn't have the tools to cope. My self-esteem took a huge beating and as a result, I felt safest at home so I stayed home all the time.

I did call the public health nurses with questions and concerns. I just wish I had the nerve to tell them what I was feeling. I was too scared, though. I didn't want Ella to be taken away. I was hoping they could sense my pain. I also felt like it was a weakness to admit that I was finding motherhood hard.

I felt like a monster. I couldn't keep my daughter happy, and I couldn't keep my husband happy. I certainly wasn't happy. I was absolutely miserable.

When Ella was eight months old, I became numb and heavy with shame and guilt. I would cry on the phone with Ward, because I was so sick and tired over Ella's crying and her not wanting to nurse and sleep. Ward finally took control and demanded I get help because he was about to have his own nervous breakdown, too.

So, I accepted my mom's offer to stay with us for a few weeks. In the meantime, I asked my doctor for help, too. I brought a list of symptoms I thought I was experiencing related to postpartum depression. My doctor decided to test my hormones and the tests came back normal. I guess I didn't have postpartum depression, and she sent me on my way.

I started to second guess myself. Maybe I don't have postpartum depression and anxiety. I did my best to cope with my feelings on my own, in my own way, and thankfully I also had the support of family and friends. As the months and years went by, I realized that I most likely did have postpartum depression and anxiety and that a hormone test probably isn't enough to rule it out one way or another. We as moms deserve better from our health-care system. I believe I should have been referred to a perinatal mental health specialist for further assessment. I'm lucky in that my depression and anxiety were mild. But what about all the other moms that fall through the cracks?

Elita Paterson is mom to Ella Bella and lives in Regina, Saskatchewan. She was instrumental in the development of the MotherFirst Report along with Dr. Angela Bowen and over 30 health-care providers. The report enabled Saskatchewan to adopt a maternal mental health strategy, one of the only provinces in Canada to have one.

HOW COMMON IS POSTPARTUM ANGER?

Christine Ou

"People say you don't know what love is until you've had a child. BS. The emotion you really don't understand until you have kids isn't love. It's rage."
-Emily Flake, New Yorker cartoonist and illustrator.

PERINATAL ANGER AND RAGE ARE the neglected mood problems of the perinatal mood and anxiety disorders (PMADs) (Ou & Hall, 2018). The transition to parenthood is filled with many emotions including joy and love, but that does not stop women from also having negative feelings. Women are given the heads-up about the baby blues and feeling out of sorts, but rarely does anyone talk about anger. Mothers have talked about how early motherhood experiences led them to feel frustrated, bad-tempered, plain angry, and even raging. It is unsurprising that some women experience anger when there are so many stressors related to the transition to parenthood for mothers. Stressors include learning how to care for a vulnerable, small human being while also meeting your own needs, and having less time for yourself and your partner, all the while dealing with the physical changes related to childbirth and breastfeeding, and lack of sleep. Studies have linked stress and lack of sleep with anger (Krizan & Hisler, 2019; Martin & Dahlen, 2005).

Anger is a fascinating emotion. Think about the last time you felt angry. How did you feel? You might have felt hot, tense or shaky, burning, or like your heart was pounding. Maybe you clenched your fist or gritted your teeth and felt like you wanted to act out in anger—maybe raise your voice, swear, or crumple that piece of paper in your hand. Sometimes anger can even make us feel out of control. What makes us feel that way and why do we get angry? Anger is an emotional reaction to a perceived harm, threat, insult, injustice, or inequality (DiGiussepe & Tafrate, 2007; Potegal, Stemmler, & Spielberger, 2010; Tavris, 1989).

Not being heard or listened to by others or encountering obstructions to your goals can also make you feel angry.

It is astonishing that anger is an emotion that we rarely acknowledge and talk about as a part of the motherhood experience. Common triggers for anger in the postpartum include but are not limited to, a traumatic birth experience, feeling like you are doing more than your fair share for the baby and at home, not being able to meet your own needs, not feeling heard by partners, family members, or health care providers, and feeling stressed and overwhelmed from having to field the needs of older little ones as well as the baby (Beck, 2002; Klein, Hyde, Essex, & Clark, 1998; Ou & Hall, 2018). Women also report feeling angry at themselves for failing to meet their expectations. The important thing about anger is that it serves as a signal to us that something is not all right.

While acknowledging that anger can cloud our thinking and prompt us to act in ways we later regret, it is important to bear in mind that anger can be an adaptive and motivating emotion that propels us to act on a situation that is unacceptable to us, whether that is through trying to constructively take control of a situation or negotiating with others (Averill, 1982). For example, merely telling someone you feel angry may prompt them to stop a problematic behavior. However, collectively we tend to be uncomfortable with anger. Society generally views anger as a conflict-causing and destructive emotion, an emotion to be avoided (Tavris, 1989). Furthermore, anger has also been socially constructed as an inappropriate emotion for women (Chemaly, 2018). Women, especially mothers, are expected to be constantly warm, loving, and nurturing (Arendell, 2010). There is a long history of disapproval about the anger of women, with disparaging labels placed on women who express anger as being "shrill" or "hysterical." Women may be more likely to develop depression because depression is a more socially acceptable way for women to express distress (Chemaly, 2018). Some emotion researchers have hypothesized that women's anger is an underlying factor behind high rates of depression for women (Asgeirsdottir & Sigfusdottir, 2015; Simon & Lively, 2010). It is hard for women to admit being angry especially when having a baby is seen as a happy and fulfilling time for women. These reasons contribute to postpartum anger being neglected as a perinatal mood problem.

How common is perinatal anger?

There are no population estimates of perinatal anger the way there are for perinatal depression and anxiety. However, some studies have suggested that anger is definitely a salient mood for some women during pregnancy and after childbirth (Bruno et al., 2017; Field, 2003; 2005; Ou & Hall, 2018). Although anger can occur on its own, often it can be associated with other emotions like guilt, hurt, sadness, shame, stress, and disappointment (Beck, 2002; Ellsworth & Tong, 2006). Not surprisingly, anger can co-occur with depression and anxiety symptoms during the perinatal period (Field et al., 2003; Kettunen, Koistinen, & Hintikka, 2014; Vliegen et al., 2013). That makes it important that we pay attention to anger. Some studies show that anger can intensify the experience of depression (Cassiello-Robbins & Barlow, 2016; Kettunen et al., 2014; Vliegen et al., 2013), making a hard situation that much harder. It is normal and human to feel anger, but if you find yourself getting angry frequently or intensely, and feeling distressed about your anger, it is important to get professional support (e.g., referrals to counseling or reproductive mental health and postpartum support groups) to help reduce the severity, frequency, and effects of anger.

What can I do about anger and rage in the moment?

Having a new baby can present stressful situations, and some mothers will encounter situations where they may feel angry. Anger can feel overwhelming, unstoppable, and difficult to ignore. Pay attention to your own signs of anger – do you feel hot, shaky, or tense? Learning to recognize these signs is important so you can start the process of coping with your anger. Luckily, anger is a transient emotion and there are some steps you can take to come down from anger so that you can avoid acting in anger. You can start with giving yourself a little space, practicing self-compassion, and reflecting on rather than ruminating on your anger.

First, give yourself space

Allow yourself the space to come down from angry feelings and, in the process, not doing harm to yourself or others. Women usually express fears about exposing their children to anger; mothers have related using 'mother sense' that allows them to act to protect their infant or child from their anger. Philosopher Seneca said that, "the greatest remedy for anger is delay". If at all possible, leave the room or situation even if it is for a few minutes to let those feelings of anger subside. Recognizing that it is not always possible to have time to yourself to cool off, you might take the baby out in the stroller for a walk as a way to get some breathing space or put on headphones to listen to music or a podcast while still being present with children.

Meet your needs

To reduce anger, self-compassion can be a very important tool. Having self-compassion is associated with lower levels of depression and anxiety in women after childbirth (Monteiro, Fonesca, Pereira, & Canavarro, 2019). You can initiate the practice of self-compassion by first identifying what your needs are and what would make you feel better physically and emotionally in the moment (Germer & Neff, 2013). Try to satisfy those needs when possible in situations where you still have to take care of little ones. It might be as small as getting something to eat and drink. Reach out to your partner, a friend, or a family member to see if they can step in and give you a break – it takes a village to raise a child. During the pandemic, it may not be possible to have another person outside of your household to help, but it can still be helpful to just even talk to another adult on the phone or to get out of the house for a walk outside with kids in tow.

Reflect and reframe

When you are able to have time to yourself, acknowledge that your emotions made sense at that time and reflect on the situation that made you feel angry. Be curious about your anger, not for the purposes of ruminating on what made you angry, but to work through your anger such as by identifying what led to the anger and to brainstorm some possible solutions for the problem that is triggering the anger. Journaling and writing can be helpful for this. For example, if you are feeling angry about not being able to sleep at night because the baby is not sleeping at night, you might do research on strategies to help your baby sleep. Or you might talk to your partner about the role they can play at nighttime to help you get more sleep, or both. You might also think about strategies to avoid situations where you are likely to become angry – this might entail planning to eat regularly to avoid being hangry or getting regular time for yourself to recharge. If you are feeling guilty about your anger, it can be helpful to reframe your thoughts about anger and to recognize that anger is an important step towards enabling you to overcome current challenges.

Practice self-forgiveness

Mothers can feel upset, guilty, and self-critical after feeling and expressing anger. Remember that having and taking care of a baby is a mentally, emotionally, and physically demanding job and that there is a lot of socio-cultural pressure on women to be a "good mother" but mothers are largely left to figure out how to mother on their own. If you are feeling angry at yourself, accept that you are only human and therefore imperfect, and talk to yourself kindly as you would talk to your child or a loved one.

In summary, parents are often unaware that they may have recurrent angry feelings during the transition to parenthood. Moreover, not all health care providers understand that anger is part of the spectrum of PMADs and or assess parents for recurrent and intense anger. Intense anger is actually a fairly common perinatal experience and there is a need to inform women, families, and clinicians about anger as a PMAD to normalize talking about postpartum anger so that parents feel comfortable getting formal and informal supports and resources to address anger and the causes of anger.

Christine Ou is a Registered Nurse, Doctoral Candidate, and Public Scholar at the University of British Columbia. Christine is also an active member of the Canadian Perinatal Mental Health Collaborative. For her dissertation, she examined maternal anger in the context of mother-infant sleep. As a UBC Public Scholar, Christine has partnered with Pacific Post Partum Support Society on projects that support postpartum parents coping with PMADs. Listen to her podcast on how to get enough sleep after having a baby: http://postpartum.org/podcast/beyond-postpartum-ep-30/ Connect with Christine on Twitter @ChristineOuBC

HONEST AS A MOTHER

Amanda Gurman

I THOUGHT POSTPARTUM DEPRESSION MEANT you were crying all the time and you have to harm yourself or your child. This is what I had been told by my doctor, my family, and society.

The day that I had my daughter was one of the happiest days of my life. She was perfect in every way, and I was so excited to have her complete our family.

The first few weeks went by and they were tough, but nothing that I had not experienced with my son.

When Scarlett was nine weeks old, my husband went back to work, and I quickly seemed to settle into the stay-at-home mom life. I was doing really great until the sleep deprivation caught up with me. I realized that I couldn't sleep when the baby was sleeping when I had a toddler running around who also needed me.

My days were long. I hated when my husband left. I felt trapped being within our home. I hated my husband for working. I was envious that he got to leave and see adults and not have to be a dad for eight hours. I pretty much started to hate everything, even being a mom.

My behaviour changed so much and so fast. I was snappy with my toddler and mean to my husband. When my daughter cried in the night for her feeding, it would enrage me. I still struggle to say that out loud. She was four months old, and I hated when she cried. *What kind of mother are you?* I would think. *Your children deserve better than you.*

These thoughts would overwhelm me more than I can ever explain. I was stuck in this vicious cycle of getting angry, screaming, feeling horrible, saying I'll do better the next day, and I wouldn't. I just continued to hate myself more and more. When Scarlett would have a bad night, I would turn it into a bad next day. I started to dread every day that I woke up.

I didn't know who I was anymore. *How did this happen to me? This is supposed to be the most exciting time of my life and I am not happy. WTF is wrong with me?* I hated my day-to-day life. I would curl up in my son's bed with him reminiscing the days of it being just him and me, and how easy it was, and how happy I was back then. I wished I could have gone back, but I couldn't. I had to fix this. My children deserved a mom who was happy. They deserved to see a mom who loved herself, so I could be a role model for them.

One day when my husband came home from work, I told him everything. I said, "I think something is wrong. I am not myself. I'm just..." and he interrupted me and quickly said, "Angry." His words cut me like a knife I couldn't believe I had become the angry mom and he could see it. I already felt like a horrible mom, but now I thought I was also a horrible wife. He told me he had seen it for weeks, but he didn't know how to help me. He suggested I call my doctor, and I did.

Within a few weeks I was seen by a mental health counsellor and it changed my perspective on everything. I learned in my first appointment that anger can represent both anxiety and depression. I had never heard of that before. This can be referred to as postpartum rage. My anger was coming from anxiety. I was feeling that so many of my needs were not met, and I was not able to control what was going on around me. I lost myself, and anger took over. I did not express that I needed help, as many of us moms do because we feel like it's our job to put others' needs ahead of our own. My counsellor taught me many ways to cope. She taught me how to calm myself down, how to express my frustrations with my children and my husband without yelling, but most importantly, she taught me how to be kind to myself during this time.

It took a long time. I stayed in therapy for just over a year, and I am still a work in progress. Alongside therapy, I found so much peace in mom blogs that I found on the Internet in the middle of the night while googling postpartum rage (which I did more often than I'd like to admit). I met some pretty amazing women on Instagram. They helped me see clearly that what I was feeling was normal. They made me see that lots of other moms go through this too and that I was not alone. With the tools that I learned in therapy and then some normalizing of my feelings with these other moms, I finally saw that it's okay to not be okay, even if you are a mom.

Amanda Gurman is a mom of two and lives in Hamilton, Ontario. Amanda is the host of a podcast called *Honest as a Mother* where she interviews other moms and experts about motherhood and perinatal mental health. You can find Amanda on Instagram @honest.as.a.mother_

THERE IS HOPE

Sara Beckel

AT TWO WEEKS POSTPARTUM, THE world around me came crashing down. Nobody told me about postpartum mental health, or at least, nobody told me about the depth of the illness in a realistic way and how it impacts absolutely everything. And lastly, nobody told me how to regain my health.

Looking back now, I can see that my decline was gradual but once it started, it took me *all* the way to the bottom. At two weeks postpartum, I was struggling with breastfeeding, and my daughter was colicky. The crying wouldn't stop and it was like my brain couldn't handle it. It felt like a short circuit. Considering I had nursed my first daughter without any major complications, this time around, I felt like a complete and utter failure. From my perspective, the one unique tool I had as a mother wasn't working and the anxiety took over.

The thing with anxiety is that it lies to you. It makes you believe you're a bad parent and that's exactly what happened to me. Nothing would soothe her. The days and nights were long and while trying to find balance within the chaos of a newborn, I was also trying to meet the needs of my toddler. To say I was in over my head was an understatement.

The weeks continued and things got worse, much, much worse. Frustration soon turned into full-blown rage, and I don't wish that on anyone. The feeling of your blood boiling in a matter of seconds is terrifying. Realizing how irrational I was with zero control over the situation was demoralizing. I remember screaming out in frustration many times throughout the day, only to be followed up with the freight train of guilt and shame that came next. It was like being on an insane roller coaster with no end in sight.

I wasn't sleeping. I was up every hour on the hour for months. Looking back now, I know how vitally important sleep is but between a toddler being up at night and a baby who nursed around the clock, sleep was nowhere to be found. I was suffering greatly and although my partner was supportive, he had no idea how to help. I remember feeling so jealous that he got to leave the house to go to work every day. I would have paid money to leave the nightmare I was living.

Months went by and I continued to get worse. Not only was I battling bouts of rage, but the depression was setting in and I could barely get out of bed. My body hurt from head to toe. I've never experienced something like that in my life. I remember having absolutely no will to move and sadly, at times, no will to live. I was just going through the motions of my day and although I knew I didn't want to die, I definitely didn't want to live like this anymore. Those were scary days that I kept to myself for the most part out of fear of losing my kids and the fear of being judged.

Finally, after six months of hell on earth, I hit a breaking point. I searched the Internet for a sliver of hope, and the more I learned about postpartum depression, the more I realized that I was in too deep and there would be no way out without support. The denial was real and it took many months of mental gymnastics trying to rationalize what was happening to me. *Maybe if I did more yoga, maybe if I ate better, maybe if I got a break, it would help?* But the fact of the matter was, I was completely paralyzed in this illness and even the simplest of self-care seemed impossible.

I eventually found a support person online. To this day, I have no idea who I called but I did have a phone call with a woman who specialized in perinatal mental health. That phone call changed everything. The relief was tremendous. I didn't have to carry this weight all by myself. She understood what this illness was. She gave me clear and tangible steps forward and above all, she gave me the hope that I so desperately needed.

Following that first conversation, I saw my naturopath because I knew I was depleted on all ends of the spectrum. She understood immediately and helped me build a basic nutritional plan. We focused on exercise and moving my body every day so I could gain strength. I eventually did some counselling as well which brought even more perspective and practical tools to reframe my thoughts.

As I began to feel better, I felt a strong pull in the direction of helping others. If this was hard for me to navigate as a fairly resourced person, how difficult must it be for people who don't have the support that I did? My experience through perinatal mental illness certainly fuelled my passion to pay it forward. As a mother of two daughters, I couldn't stand the fact that it could be the same for them when they grow up. I couldn't stand the fact that it was so hard to find resources. And if it wasn't me contributing to changing it, then who would?

This journey, although excruciating at times, has taught me some of the best and most important lessons of my life. It's taught me unconditional love. It's taught me self-compassion and that prioritizing my needs first is the best way to take care of my family. Above all, it has connected me with mom, parents, and advocates all across North America. Being part of this perinatal community has brought me so much healing and happiness that I could have never envisioned during those early weeks of my postpartum journey.

If you're reading this now, in the heat of a perinatal mental illness, I want you to know you're not alone. There is help, and of course, there is hope.

Sara Beckel is a mom of two and lives in Regina, Saskatchewan. She is proud to be recognized as Regina's "Best Doula" through *Prairie Dog Magazine's* annual campaign and was named as a 2019 CBC Future 40 Recipient. Sara launched a new initiative called the Regina Perinatal Health Network (RPHN), which offers free perinatal support within the community.

Part 4:

Postpartum Bipolar Disorder & Postpartum Psychosis

CRACKED

And then I cracked.
Like furrows of dried plaster.
Before immaculately seamless,
Now a silhouette of mountains
Foreboding; fearful apprehension.

It doesn't weaken me.
My structural integrity is still unbroken
But I see it every day.
I know it is there.
I anticipate its expansion.

But this time others can see it.
Comforted to know that they can recognise it.

We're maintaining vigilance.

Leander Moore
@Postpartumpoet

MANIC MOM

Patricia Tomasi

I SPENT WEEKS FEELING DEPRESSED and hopeless following the birth of my first daughter when one morning, seemingly out of the blue, I woke up full of energy and went about my day like the Energizer bunny. I wouldn't stop. I couldn't stop. I felt like a new person, like I was superhuman.

I also had all these ideas firing into my head that I desperately needed to get down on paper before they evaporated into the ether from whence they came. I thought I was solving life's biggest riddles. I felt as though I was chosen to receive a download of information from the universe, which I scrambled to scribble down on whatever bits of napkin and torn pieces of paper I could find.

What was happening to me? Unfortunately, it would take eight years before learning that in those early days of feeling otherworldly and in the months that ensued, I was suffering from a manic episode due to unscreened, unassessed, and untreated postpartum bipolar disorder.

The psychosis came next.

Over the coming days and weeks, I filled notebooks of thoughts. I was ecstatic that the depression I had been living with since labour had finally lifted and that I suddenly felt so good inside instead of so terrible.

It's gone, I kept thinking. *The postpartum depression is gone!*

I mean, I thought it was postpartum depression. Up to that point, I hadn't been diagnosed or anything. I did score high on the Edinburgh Postnatal Depression Scale that day I called the public health nurse. She came over and sat on my couch for an hour and told me to get more sleep and meditate so I assumed that meant I was suffering from some form of postpartum depression. Or maybe it was the baby blues? She never did tell me to get a proper assessment. Take a walk, take a break, you'll feel better, is all she said. No talk of prior mental health issues or perinatal mental health at all in fact. The same held true for my six-week postpartum check up at the obstetrician's office which lasted all of five minutes.

Well that was all in the past now because as of that manic morning, I felt on top of the world! *Guess meditation really did the trick,* I thought. It was supposed to calm me down and put me back in the moment but unfortunately, it did more than that for me. I started imagining all these places in my mind that I thought were real. I started to think it was enabling me to tap into a special frequency and give me a direct channel to God. I started to believe it had cured me of postpartum depression.

Not only was I not depressed, I was the extreme opposite of depressed. I was euphoric. I was high. It felt like I was being fed a constant source of energy that was feeding my veins. I felt limitless.

I thought I was happy but what I really was, was impatient and irritated. I needed to get things done, so many things and everyone and everything around me moved at a pace much too slow for my new super brain. If you weren't as jubilated and excited about new age spirituality as I was right now, then you needed to get out of my way. I didn't have time for a husband who was deeply confused with my beliefs or a baby that was always needing my attention. I had advanced spiritually, and they just needed to keep up.

Did I mention I suddenly had so many things to do? God, angels, spirit guides, and aliens on the Orion belt were communicating with me through secret coded messages on licence plates and billboards. They told me I was one of the chosen ones sent to earth to reawaken humanity. I had a mission to fulfill, and I needed to get on it stat! I needed to tell other moms that meditation was the cure for postpartum depression, I needed to quit my job to become a Reiki master and chakra healer, and lastly, I needed to fulfill my childhood dream of becoming a famous actor.

This new me was intoxicating.

I started to see auras of colour emanating from people's bodies and felt I could interpret what it meant. Glowing yellow? You were too cerebral today. Try focusing on your heart chakra. Glowing blue? You're speaking your truth. Black? Oh oh...better get yourself to a doctor, or better yet, here, take these crystals and place them on your third eye. That will help.

I thought I had been granted special healing powers. I bought a massage table and started bringing strangers into my home for hands-on healing sessions. I also had to constantly cleanse my home with smoky sage to get rid of the demon shadows I could see floating around the ceiling.

Besides delusions of grandeur, hallucinations, and strange new beliefs centred around spirituality, I also started spending money, lots of it. I dropped thousands of dollars on new age courses and trainings and certifications and conferences and books and a *magic* dragon ring that I thought could enhance my powers (that ring was $2000 alone).

I self-published a book within the span of a week, which I'm still trying to desperately wipe from the Internet. It's part memoir, part guide book on how to manifest your *kick ass dreams* through balancing your chakras. (I was obsessed with chakras.)

My mania and psychosis reached its peak at a book launch I planned to coincide with Bell Let's Talk Day in 2013. I was, after all, raising awareness of the magic of meditation and postpartum depression, which I believed was part of my special earthly purpose.

It didn't help that I had friends in high places in the media world who were more than willing to join me on this fantastic voyage. Believe it or not, (I still can't), I managed to get a two-page spread in the *Toronto Sun*. There I was in a full-on Mariah Carey, diva-esque pose, sequined outfit and all next to an article about a woman who had bravely quit her job to follow her dreams. That woman was me. Why the *Toronto Sun* decided to print that article is beyond me.

I guess I was also really good at convincing people that what I was saying about moms and mental health and the universe and following your dreams was all real, because I truly believed it. Though friends and strangers maybe joked about how psychotic I was acting behind my back, the truth is, I really was, and needed help.

I don't blame my friends and family for not staging an intervention. I wouldn't have listened to them anyway. Besides, I wasn't hurting anyone, not in the obvious physical sense. So what if I was a little out there and eccentric? The mania was making me fun again after being such a drag for so long. I was like a circus freak. Who wouldn't want tickets to that sideshow?

To make matters worse, I got a call from CTV news channel asking me to appear live on their national morning show on Bell Let's Talk Day to talk about my book and postpartum journey. It was just more confirmation for me that I was doing God's work.

When veteran anchors, Dan Matheson and Jacqueline Milczarek, asked me about my postpartum depression experience, this is what I said: "I believe it was more of an existential crisis more than anything... and it's the chakra system and meditation that cured me."

Oh cringe. Facepalm and cringe.

If only I could go back and tell everyone not to listen to me, that I was suffering and manic, and that if screening for perinatal mental health existed then (or now), maybe I wouldn't be on this national television show spewing incorrect information to vulnerable moms at home.

That night, friends and strangers showed up to my book launch, which consisted of me performing a one-woman musical all about my journey in an actual theatre I dropped thousands more to rent out for the evening. And yes, it was as ridiculous as it sounds. I changed the words to Michael Jackson songs and the theme from *The Little Mermaid* and told my story of how the chakras cured me. I actually ended up raising $1000 through ticket sales, which I donated to a mental health charity, so at least some good came out of that bewildering time.

But I reached the peak of my manic journey and was about to fall, hard. Just before I hit bottom, I became pregnant again, and I credit the rising hormones and the sedating effect they had on my neurotransmitters for saving me.

After I gave birth to my second daughter, I skipped the depression part and went straight to euphoria. But three months later, instead of the manic high I began experiencing after the birth of my first daughter, things got dark, really dark. I started having intrusive thoughts, flashes of terrifying images like driving off a cliff with my baby or watching her drown in a bathtub. I felt like I was drifting further and further from reality as each day passed. It was like I was there, but I wasn't. Things and people started feeling far away from me. I was catatonic. I would stare at the wall all day. I started experiencing derealization, depersonalizaton, and awful, awful panic attacks. This time, I wasn't going to end up in a sparkly dress on stage performing to an audience of well-wishers. This time, I really feared I could end up dead.

Somehow, to this day, I don't know why or how, but I had enough awareness and wherewithal to haul ass into my doctor's office and demand medication. I had actually started reading about perinatal mental health during pregnancy as I moved further away from mania and closer to lucidity and began to realize that I had probably experienced a severe perinatal mental illness. So I guess my guard was up and I was able to notice things were taking a very wrong turn and that I needed help. Fast.

And thank God, not the God I thought I could communicate with during my manic, psychotic episode, but thank the figurative, questionable, and elusive God, the medication worked. Within six weeks, I started feeling like myself again and within a few months, I had felt the sanest I had ever felt in my life. I got to enjoy motherhood and my daughter got all of my attention. I loved her to bits and doted on her day and night. I felt like I managed to jump off the spinning wheel I was stuck on. For years.

"Didn't anyone find your behaviour a little odd?" asked the psychiatrist eight years after my postpartum bipolar manic psychotic episode. (Try saying that ten times fast.)

I know what you're thinking. Eight years?? Why did it take so long? It's because I finally managed to get a referral to the Women's College Hospital Life Stages Reproductive Program in Toronto, one of the only specialist perinatal mental health programs in the country. Though I was way past the referral time frame of one-year postpartum, I was able to get in on account of the fact that I was concerned about the next potentially mental health disruptive reproductive stage in my life, menopause.

But really, I was there to get answers about what had happened to me all those years ago.

"Yes, I think so, but no one said anything, at least, not to my face," I tell her. "I was always known for being silly and spontaneous, except when I was really depressed. It's funny how I had all these ups and downs during childhood and adolescence. And then in my twenties I started having panic attacks but even though I tried to get help, I was given the runaround by the health care system and was never able to get a proper assessment."

"Sounds like you had anxiety and depression growing up, which may have actually been bipolar disorder," she said. "Any mental health condition puts you at a higher risk of developing a perinatal mental illness. And I'm sure what you experienced was postpartum bipolar disorder with mania and psychosis. You should have been flagged and treated."

I felt relieved to finally have some answers and even start putting the pieces together of different times in my life when I now know I wasn't crazy or being difficult or selfish in my unending sadness. I was fucking suffering from mental health conditions I needed help for!

It's true that no one got hurt, physically. But I did end up losing my house after spending all my savings, my career after angels told me to quit my job, and almost my marriage were it not for my understanding husband. I also very dangerously spread a very incorrect message to moms suffering from postpartum depression. Meditation and the chakras cannot cure postpartum depression. Probably, the biggest regret I have today about the fallout from my untreated postpartum bipolar disorder is the effect it might have had on my daughter's own mental health.

She's a wonderful 11-year-old girl today with an awesome sense of humour and quirkiness about her we all love, but she was also diagnosed with Attention Deficit Hyperactivity Disorder, Autism, Tourette's Syndrome, and anxiety at age six. Did my illness play any part in that? Will she struggle with her mental health as she gets older or one day becomes a mom herself? Interestingly, my second daughter who is six today, has none of the mental health issues my first daughter has. Is that because I was treated in a timely manner? These thoughts play heavily on my mind.

A book I read during my healing journey really had me understand the science behind perinatal mental health and that I was suffering from a physical, biological illness. It was an epiphany. The book was *This Isn't What I Expected* by Karen Kleiman. How amazing to have Karen part of this anthology I dreamed of creating for moms. I feel like I've come full circle.

I started openly talking about my discoveries and experiences on social media and sparking a lot of conversation between my mom friends on Facebook. One of those friends was an editor at *HuffPost Canada* and she asked if I wanted to start blogging about it for them. I jumped at the chance to tell the right story this time. I quickly became *HuffPost Canada's* perinatal mental health journalist and started exposing how far behind Canada was in universal screening and treatment and mother and baby units of which Canada still has not-a-one.

In 2019, I decided to make the leap from journalist to full time advocate and formed the Canadian Perinatal Mental Health Collaborative along with Jaime Charlebois, Ontario's only Perinatal Mental Health Mood Disorder coordinator whom I had interviewed for one of my *HuffPost* articles. She, too, experienced perinatal mental illness and a lack of support and she, too, decided to devote her efforts towards changing the system. In two short years, we have put together a team of experts from across Canada who are helping us lobby the government for a national perinatal mental health strategy and we won't stop until we get it.

This isn't just a health issue, this is a rights issue. Moms and people everywhere across Canada deserve to have timely access to the best specialist perinatal mental health treatment should they so need it. There's nothing less at stake than the mental well-being of the next generation.

Patricia Tomasi is a mom of two from Barrie, Ontario. She is a former-journalist-turned-fierce-advocate for perinatal mental health. She went from writing about maternal mental health for *HuffPost Canada* to co-founding the Canadian Perinatal Mental Health Collaborative and lobbying the federal government for a national perinatal mental health strategy. Connect with Patricia on Instagram @maternal_mental_health_matters and on Twitter @PatriciaVTomasi

TOTALLY UNEXPECTED

Geneviève Desrochers

My pregnancy came as a surprise, four months after marriage. It was a beautiful surprise as both my husband and I were thrilled. But I also felt nervous.

Will I be a good mom? Will I know how to best take care of my baby? Will I be able to make him happy? Will he grow up to be a responsible person?

I wanted to do everything in my power to prepare myself for what I considered to be the beginning of a new and important journey for us. I started to plan and read about pregnancy, labour, and breastfeeding. I bought baby clothes and baby gear, and I took a prenatal class with my husband.

We chose to labour at home with midwives. We were excited and felt confident about this decision. We did everything in our knowledge to get ready for the arrival of our son.

But one thing I did not pay much attention to was educating myself about postpartum mental health.

The prenatal workshop facilitator did cover the subject and spoke about the baby blues and depression, but there was not much time spent on it. As I was listening to this part of the class, I remember telling myself that I would probably not be affected by a mental health issue in the postpartum period. Not me, with the great support I would get from my husband and all the preparation we were doing.

I was wrong.

Our son was born at the hospital after a very long and difficult birth. Our dreams of a home birth did not come true. I was exhausted and disappointed but also happy to finally be able to hold my baby in my arms.

In the weeks that followed, I lived on cloud nine. I was experiencing the happiest time of my life and savoring every minute of our new family reality. What I did not realize though was that my mood was abnormally high. Despite the enormous lack of sleep, I did not feel the need to rest during the day and properly sleep during the night, between feeds. Instead, I would find myself writing long emails to friends, posting on Facebook and even writing a children's story in the wee hours of the night. My mind was flooded with ideas that I absolutely needed to put down on paper.

After three weeks of this very exhilarating way of living, I entered a new phase that started to worry my husband. I started feeling tired finally, but was still unable to sleep when I wanted to. I started having delusions about my husband dying every time he would go out for errands and I was convinced that God was guiding me to prevent a horrible event that would happen to my sister. I was listening to what I thought was an order, direct from the Holy Spirit and wrote my sister a long email in the middle of the night that I thought would save her.

There was also an excruciating pain in my right leg that would keep me awake during the night and cause me to limp during the day. I thought I had a blood clot in my thigh when I was in fact experiencing a tactile hallucination.

I started to experience terrifying panic attacks, and my husband had no clue what was going on with me.

We called my midwife and were able to see her shortly after. She told us to go straight to the emergency room. One month after the birth of our son, I was admitted to hospital not knowing that I was in the middle of a manic episode with psychotic symptoms. I had no clue what was happening to me.

One day later, after a series of physical tests, a doctor told me that I would be sent home the following day if the ultrasound done on my right thigh came back normal. There was no screening done and no questions asked regarding my mental health. We could hardly believe it. By now, my husband and I knew there was something wrong with me, something regarding my mental health.

My midwife came to visit me, and I told her what was happening. She put us in touch with a social worker who contacted a great psychiatrist at the hospital who came to see me. I stayed in the hospital for about a week. After a few sessions with the psychiatrist, I received the diagnosis of bipolar disorder of postpartum onset with psychotic features. This was a diagnosis that was totally unexpected. I had no symptoms prior to birth and no history of this mental illness in my family. What a shock!

I'll never forget the days after I received my medication for the first time, when that little pill I was swallowing started to calm my ill brain. A grieving process was starting. At first, there was that one big scary question that was haunting me: *Will I ever be myself again or will I be comfortable with who I will become?* I wished so hard that things would go back to normal quickly. I soon realized that it would take some time. I had to take one day, one moment at a time.

Beyond that fear, something else emerged unexpectedly—a new passion was born in me. At that moment, I knew deep down in my heart, that one day I would use my experience to help future and new parents. I would tell my story, share the knowledge I gained about postpartum mood and anxiety disorders, and find a way to inform and support parents if they found themselves going through a similar challenge. I would do my best to try to erase the stigma still attached to postpartum mental illnesses.

My recovery process was challenging, and I did experience depression a couple months after my manic episode. I was losing interest in my son and felt like I did not deserve to be his mom. Everything felt like a burden. But thankfully, with antidepressants and the amazing support of my psychiatrist, my husband, family members, and friends, in time, I was able to recover and feel like myself again.

Geneviève Desrochers is a postpartum doula and lives in Brampton with her two kids and husband. Hear her tell her story in her own words in French and English on her YouTube channel and find her on Instagram @transition_postpartum_support.

POSTPARTUM BIPOLAR DISORDER

Dr. Verinder Sharma and Dr. Michael Thomson

BIPOLAR DISORDER IS NOT A single entity but rather a group of conditions including bipolar I disorder, bipolar II disorder, and other specified bipolar and related disorder. A diagnosis of bipolar I disorder requires at least one manic episode, however, the majority of individuals also have periods of major depression. Bipolar II disorder is characterized by episodes of hypomania as well as major depression. The other specified bipolar and related disorder is generally considered a catch-all category for cases of bipolar disorder that do not meet the diagnostic criteria for bipolar I or II disorder.

During mania, the mood is abnormally and persistently happy or irritable, and the individual has increased energy for a period of at least one week (or any duration if hospital admission is necessary). In addition there are symptoms such as feelings of great importance or increased self-esteem, decreased need for sleep, talkativeness, racing thoughts or flight of ideas, poor judgment, and impulsive behavior. Hypomania has similar symptoms but they are less severe, and are of shorter duration (at least 4 days).

During depression, the mood is abnormally sad or indifferent for at least two weeks, and there are other symptoms such as appetite change causing weight loss or weight gain, sleep change in the form of insomnia (trouble falling asleep and/or staying asleep), or hypersomnia (sleeping too much), loss of energy, guilt, poor concentration, agitation or being slowed down physically and mentally, as well as suicidal thoughts. Bipolar disorder is often accompanied by other psychiatric disorders such as substance use disorder, anxiety disorders, or obsessive-compulsive disorder.

Bipolar I disorder is equally common in men and women while bipolar II disorder appears to be more common in women. Bipolar disorder usually begins during late adolescence or early adulthood. In women the disorder tends to cluster during the childbearing years as some women have onset of symptoms around puberty or following childbirth while others have worsening of symptoms before menstrual periods or around menopause. What causes bipolar disorder is not fully understood. Various reproductive events such as puberty, menstrual periods, pregnancy and menopause influence the course of bipolar disorder but none as dramatically as the postpartum period. Thus hormonal changes play a role in the onset or aggravation of symptoms of bipolar disorder. A family history of bipolar disorder also increases the risk of developing bipolar disorder. Sleep loss—a common occurrence after childbirth-can also trigger mood and psychotic episodes in some women.

Postpartum mood disorders

Mood disorders in the postpartum period have traditionally been thought to include the baby blues, postpartum depression and postpartum psychosis. The baby blues affect 30 to 75% of women during the first few days after childbirth. The usual symptoms include sadness, tearfulness, irritability, frequent mood changes and poor sleep. The symptoms typically begin within three to four days and disappear by the tenth day after delivery. As the symptoms are usually mild and time-limited, no treatment is required. However, the symptoms persist and can develop into an episode of postpartum depression or postpartum psychosis in some women. It is currently unknown how common the baby blues are in women with bipolar disorder.

Few people are aware that baby pinks are also common after delivery. The term baby pinks is used to describe symptoms such as elation, over talkativeness, feeling more active than usual, decreased need for sleep, feelings of being an important person, racing thoughts and distractibility. The symptoms appear immediately after delivery and don't last for more than a few days. In most cases no treatment is required. However, these symptoms are the first manifestation of bipolar disorder in some women. There is also growing evidence that a variety of other psychiatric disorders such as obsessive-compulsive disorder or anxiety disorders can recur or begin for the first time after delivery. As the following case illustrates the first onset of these disorders in the postpartum period places women at high risk of developing bipolar disorder in the future.

After my son was born at the end of 2007, I was diagnosed with postpartum obsessive-compulsive disorder a couple of months later. I had heard about depression, but no one warned me of this illness. I felt lost, and my intrusive and obsessive thoughts were out of control. By spring, my doctor put me on Zoloft, which kept the OCD at bay until my daughter was born during the summer of 2010. Once my little one was born, I felt immensely different. I entered into a very deep depression. My relationship with my daughter was suffering as, I could find no joy in parenthood - or in anything for that matter. Once I was put on Abilify, with the Zoloft, I felt some relief. I stayed on this combination until the spring of 2014. At this time, I had begun to notice a big shift in my behavior. I had noticeable periods where I was awake for at least days at a time. I didn't do much about this at the time because to be honest I loved the energy, efficiency, and euphoria I felt. I ignored the increased moments of agitation, because I was living in an immense high. However, I was exhibiting a complete lack of control over my impulses. I became hypersexual putting many at risk. By the end of June, my brain had become so chaotic, that I couldn't tell if I was high or extremely sad. I wouldn't admit that anything was wrong until my suicidal thoughts literally had me trying to form the right words to put into my kids' goodbye letters. I was at work one afternoon, and I was compelled to go to a friend for help, she took me to the hospital, where I stayed for 3 weeks after being diagnosed with bipolar disorder. I disliked being in the hospital, but I finally found some relief. With the right medications, I have been able to live a normal life. I do have my cycles, but they are more predictable and manageable. Not a day goes by that I don't wish my illness away, but I am truly thankful for my medical and familial support.

Childbirth and bipolar disorder

The postpartum period has long been recognized as a time of increased risk for recurrence of mood episodes in women with bipolar disorder. In one study more than 50% of women with bipolar I or II disorder had an episode of major depression, hypomania, mania, or anxiety during the first six months after delivery. Symptoms of bipolar postpartum depression are similar to symptoms of bipolar depression at other times with a few exceptions.

During the postpartum period women may have obsessive worries about the well-being of the newborn or have a fear of harming the baby. Women feel overwhelmed due to the stress of providing care to their children. The postpartum period is also a high-risk time for the occurrence of hypomanic, manic or psychotic episodes. It is unclear how common mania is after delivery because a large number of women with mania may be diagnosed as having postpartum psychosis.

Typically, postpartum psychosis or mania are more likely to occur soon after delivery while episodes of depression can happen at any time during the postpartum period. Postpartum psychosis is the most serious psychiatric illness following childbirth and it occurs in 0.1 to 0.2% of cases. The symptoms can appear as early as 48-72 hours but usually occur during the first two weeks after childbirth. The early symptoms are rather vague and may include insomnia, agitation, and irritability. As the illness evolves, patients develop rapidly changing moods, confusion, bizarre behavior, auditory hallucinations, and delusions. The intensity of symptoms fluctuates and there may be brief periods when the individual appears free of psychiatric symptoms.

Postpartum psychosis is generally considered a mixed or manic episode of bipolar disorder, however, a depressive episode with psychosis can also present as postpartum psychosis. Because postpartum psychosis may affect decision-making ability, women may think that there is nothing wrong with them and refuse psychiatric treatment. First-time mothers, women with a history of bipolar I disorder or postpartum psychosis, and those with a family history of bipolar I disorder or postpartum psychosis are at a high risk of experiencing a psychotic episode after childbirth. Sleep loss, which is quite common around the time of delivery, is also a powerful trigger of postpartum psychosis. Some physical diseases such as thyroid disorders and certain prescription medications may cause or worsen postpartum psychosis. Postpartum psychosis is considered a psychiatric emergency and it usually requires hospitalization as the woman is at a significantly increased risk of harming herself or her children. Some women who have had postpartum psychosis will not experience another episode or will only have episodes during the postpartum period whereas others will experience episodes at other times of their life.

Relationship between postpartum depression and bipolar disorder

Postpartum depression is generally defined as occurrence of a depressive episode in the first four weeks after delivery, however, mothers remain at risk for depression for several months. Postpartum depression is either an episode of major depressive disorder (also referred to as unipolar postpartum depression) or bipolar disorder (also known as bipolar postpartum depression).

Symptoms of bipolar postpartum depression are the same as those of unipolar postpartum depression, however, women with the bipolar type are more likely to have mixed symptoms (symptoms of hypomania or mania and depression occurring together), psychotic features, and atypical symptoms (e.g. increased appetite or increased sleep requirement). In a study from the USA approximately 14% of women had postpartum depression of which nearly a quarter had bipolar disorder. In psychiatric settings over 21% to 54% of women presenting with postpartum depression meet the diagnostic criteria for bipolar disorder.

Women with more severe depression in the postpartum period are more likely to have a diagnosis of bipolar disorder. Risk factors for bipolar postpartum depression include; younger age, unplanned pregnancy, bipolar symptoms prior to pregnancy, family history of bipolar disorder, and onset of depression immediately after delivery. Women with bipolar II disorder appear to be at a particularly high risk to experience postpartum depression. As the following case illustrates, having the first onset of depression after delivery puts women at risk for developing bipolar disorder in the future.

Ms. A, a 22-year-old female became depressed for the first time within a few days of delivering her first child. She consulted her family physician who diagnosed her with major depressive disorder and initiated a trial of citalopram 20 mg daily. Within a few days she became unresponsive and stopped talking. She was admitted to hospital where she spent the next 7 months. After failing to respond to trials of various antidepressants alone or in combination with drugs from other classes she finally responded to quetiapine monotherapy. Quetiapine was stopped one year later at her request to allow her to have a medication free pregnancy. Quetiapine restarted before delivery was effective in preventing mood or psychotic episodes after the birth of her other two children. Six years after her third delivery she had a manic episode. The diagnosis was changed to bipolar I disorder and she was treated with lithium and quetiapine.

Screening and monitoring

Despite being referred to as postpartum episodes, mood disorders and psychotic episodes identified during the postpartum period sometimes start during pregnancy. Therefore, women with bipolar disorder or those who are at risk of developing the disorder should be identified as soon as possible in pregnancy. Health care providers use questionnaires such as the Mood Disorder Questionnaire (MDQ) or the Hypomania Checklist-32 to identify women with bipolar disorder. It is also important that family doctors, obstetricians, midwives and other individuals providing pregnancy care ask women if they have experienced any past mental health concerns or if anyone in their family has experienced a significant mental illness. Women identified as having bipolar disorder or being at risk for developing bipolar disorder should be referred to a psychiatrist for further assessment and treatment.

It can be challenging to identify a postpartum depressive episode that is part of a bipolar disorder rather than major depressive disorder. Likewise, it can be difficult to distinguish between the normal joys that can follow childbirth, and mild hypomanic symptoms. Health care providers, even those working within the mental health field, often get little education on postpartum bipolar disorders. As a result, misdiagnosis of bipolar postpartum depression is common and it often leads to delays in women receiving appropriate treatment.

Women with bipolar disorder should be encouraged to monitor symptoms using a mood diary or an app and to review this information on a regular basis with their health care provider. Collateral information from the spouse or another family member can be vital for identifying mood episodes early and initiating timely treatment. Suicide risk assessments are an important component of providing ongoing care to postpartum women with bipolar disorder.

Women should also be asked if they are experiencing any thoughts of harming the child or of harming anyone else. This becomes increasingly important in episodes of postpartum psychosis as the risk of homicidal behaviors is significantly higher. Intrusive thoughts or images of harming the infant are common in obsessive-compulsive disorder, however, mothers with obsessive-compulsive disorder find them distressing and attempt to suppress the thoughts. In most instances the mother will be fearful of discussing these thoughts as they worry about negative judgements or triggering an investigation by child protective services. It can be beneficial to discuss with women that these intrusive thoughts are common occurrences in women experiencing postpartum mental distress. Discussing this helps reduce mental health stigma and it allows the women to discuss her concerns with greater ease.

Treatment considerations

Education aimed at enhancing an individual's understanding of bipolar disorder, reviewing the importance of self-monitoring of symptoms, teaching effective prevention strategies, and discussing the pros and cons of different treatment approaches should be the cornerstones of the overall management plan. Since childbirth is a potent and specific trigger of hypomanic or manic episodes, the postpartum period provides a remarkable opportunity for prevention or early intervention in women at risk of developing bipolar disorder. In particular, women that have a close family member with bipolar disorder should be under the care of a psychiatrist to allow for close monitoring during pregnancy and at least into the early postpartum period.

Medications started during or after pregnancy are often effective in reducing the risk of relapse. Among mood stabilizers lithium is the most studied drug in the prevention of postpartum mood or psychotic episodes. In contrast, valproic acid is not effective in preventing mood episodes in patients with bipolar disorder. There is limited evidence that olanzapine and quetiapine may be effective in reducing the risk of relapse. Lamotrigine is effective in preventing episodes during pregnancy in women with bipolar disorder, however, it is unclear whether the medication is also effective for prevention of postpartum episodes.

Several medications are available for treatment of mania or psychosis; however, some women may refuse treatment because she cannot recognize that she is experiencing a manic or psychotic episode. Treatment of bipolar depression in the postpartum period can be challenging. Although antidepressants are commonly recommended for unipolar postpartum depression, they have not been specifically studied in women with bipolar postpartum depression. Moreover, antidepressants themselves carry a risk of inducing hypomania or mania in some women Treatment with lithium, quetiapine, lamotrigine or lurasidone should be considered in women who have a severe episode of major depression and who are at high risk of developing mania.

Those with a history of safe and effective use of an antidepressant may benefit from a retrial of the same or a similar drug. The compatibility of the medication with breastfeeding should be ensured in nursing mothers. While breastfeeding is beneficial for both the mother and the newborn, it should be discouraged in mothers with mania or psychosis. Electroconvulsive therapy (ECT) is generally reserved for patients with severe agitation, catatonia (lack of movement and communication), psychotic symptoms, or refusal to eat or drink. Similar to the lack of studies on the use of medications, there are no well-done studies on the role of psychotherapy in the treatment of bipolar postpartum depression. Interpersonal psychotherapy, an effective treatment for unipolar postpartum depression, should be considered for women who are breastfeeding or those who refuse drug treatment.

In summary, women are at an exceptionally high risk of developing or having a recurrence of bipolar disorder after delivery. First occurrence of some other psychiatric disorders in the postpartum period also increases the risk of these women developing bipolar disorder at a later date. Early identification of women with bipolar disorder or those at risk of developing the disorder is important for initiating timely and appropriate treatment. Due to the high risk of psychiatric hospitalization and safety concerns about the mother or the newborn, it is important that women be screened for bipolar disorder when they present for health care during or after pregnancy. While efforts to increase awareness of depression during and after pregnancy are laudable, let's not forget that women with a positive screen for depression also need to be screened and assessed for bipolar disorder. Unfortunately, a large number of women don't receive a correct diagnosis of, or appropriate treatment for bipolar disorder until after having children. Thus, the postpartum period provides a unique opportunity for health care professionals to play an important role in the detection, diagnosis and treatment of bipolar disorder.

Dr. Verinder Sharma graduated in medicine from Punjabi University in India, and completed his residency in psychiatry at University of Saskatchewan, Saskatoon. He is a professor of psychiatry and has a cross appointment to the department of Obstetrics & Gynecology at University of Western Ontario, London, Ontario. Currently, he is a consultant psychiatrist in the ambulatory program at Parkwood Institute, London, Ontario Dr. Sharma's research focuses on the diagnosis and treatment of refractory mood disorders and peripartum psychiatric illnesses. He is a member of the Canadian Network for Mood and Anxiety Treatments (CANMAT) as well as the International Society for Bipolar Disorders (ISBD) Women's Health task force.

Dr. Michael Thomson is a consultant psychiatrist in the ambulatory program at Parkwood Institute in London, Ontario. He completed an Honours Bachelor's degree in medical sciences with a specialization in physiology and pharmacology at the University of Western Ontario. Following this, he obtained his Doctor of Medicine (MD) degree and completed a residency in psychiatry through the Schulich School of Medicine & Dentistry at the University of Western Ontario. He is a Fellow of the Royal College of Physicians and Surgeons of Canada and an assistant professor in the Department of Psychiatry at the University of Western Ontario.His clinical work predominantly involves the treatment of chronic mood and psychotic disorders.

THIS WON'T GO BACK TO NORMAL

Holly P

I GAVE THEM A WARNING. I knew this could happen. A relative's recent psychosis meant I knew the signs, symptoms and drab psychiatric ward walls. I warned my midwife of my increased risk. She didn't seem concerned.

I am seven months pregnant when the global pandemic hits. Immediately, my husband and I lose our jobs in a decimated industry. We are packed and about to move to an apartment we can no longer afford. So we cancel moving to a bigger space and unpack back into our studio apartment.

We see no one and go nowhere. I have virtual pregnancy groups and a cancelled baby shower. I ugly cry on the phone to Amazon's customer service because they cannot deliver crib sheets until after my due date. Everything feels impossible.

My beautiful son arrives, and I have laboured for 38 hours without sleep. We're transferred to recovery and go to bed. Except I don't. I force my brain awake. Part adrenaline of birth, part unrelenting anxiety, and perhaps, already partly dipping into mania.

On the third day of not sleeping, I come undone. I obsess with tracking feedings and dirty diapers. I stare at the clock, and my brain is invaded by a dreamscape that opens a door, invites me in, and tells me, *This is psychosis.* I enter thinking, *I can do anything for one second. I can be in psychosis for one second.* So I transcend reality. I obsess with the clock, I manically scribble words trying to find the meaning of life, to crack the code. There are pyramids and rules of being a good person, and my final conclusion: Time is an illusion. In my mania, I do not see Robin or Wyatt or my hospital surroundings. I do not hear these voices. I create these voices, I am these voices. I jump into swimming through my own mind and these discoveries of delusion.

Smells, tastes, visual stimuli, and pain are the only things that pull me out of my manic mind and ground me in reality forming memories.

Flashes of eating a spicy tuna roll, my painful postpartum bowel movement, and Robin peering over me in an ambulance.

I'm at a new hospital, in a new room, and alone. I look down at my wristband and see my birthday. My brain jumps to the conclusion: That date must be the present day. I think I am my mother and I have just given birth to me. I keep writing, piecing together psychosis, the meaning of life, my brain, and time. I feel euphoric, but I know something is wrong. I tell the psychiatrist I don't care about a diagnosis or what medications I need—just fix me.

I start to come to. Many times a minute, my mind cycles through a battle of screaming, *Wake up Holly, you're in psych ward, snap out of it,* versus my airy, carefree elation. I have the wherewithal to pump. I am even more obsessed with time because of this. I can't forget to pump, I can't forget my baby.

It's been six days since I gave birth, and I have not showered. I use the washroom and notice my pad is absolutely rancid. I smell. I ask to take a shower. My day nurse gets me a towel and unlocks the shower. I turn the tap to hot water and jump in, but the water is ice cold. Everything I tell my brain to do results in the opposite happening; I am broken. I open my shower kit, and I don't know what to do. My brain is grinding and sputtering. *Wash your hair.* I dig around my shower kit and grab a shampoo-looking bottle, pour some into my hands, and scrub my hair, but it's conditioner. I use a lavender soap that I've never seen before. The smell jolts me to reality. I internally scream, *Holly, you're in a shower! What do you do in the shower?* It doesn't help. I'm too foggy. I stop my pitiful half-shower, half-done and realize I only have one small towel and dirty clothes to get to my room with.

I am so happy when Wyatt and Robin show up. I pirouette around the room instead of holding my baby. Wyatt needs a diaper change so I volunteer, but I also don't remember how. Robin repeats the steps with me, but I get distracted and leave the job half done. I daydream about going on my first walk with Wyatt outside; there are no day or overnight passes because of the pandemic. Robin suggests a slightly different walk. I walk proudly down the halls of the psychiatric ward. Wyatt receives compliments from patients and nurses alike.

It has been twelve days since giving birth. I realize Robin and Wyatt are leaving for the day and I cannot. The exit door locks. I try pulling it open but it won't budge. I find my day nurse and bother her incessantly about leaving. I know who I am, I know where I am, and I just want to go home. The next day, I'm questioned by my psychiatrist as to why I acted out. I have no explanation. I tell him I am afraid of forgetting Robin and Wyatt. He is crestfallen and shocked that could even be a worry of mine. How could that be so surprising? I have lost a full week of my life to this, lost my mind, and lost my freedom. Comparatively, losing people seems easy.

By the weekend I am getting better. I don't have a vacant stare, I converse politely with nurses, and can brush my teeth. On Sunday I have my best day yet. The sun is shining through a plexiglass window. Robin is asleep in the hospital bed, and I am sitting, holding Wyatt. I am peaceful and don't need to get up. I am there for him. I sing to him under my breath. I once again carry my baby boy.

On Tuesday, I'm finally released. I'm followed by two outpatient psychiatrists and a caseworker. I'm still not a hundred percent me. I can't read and retain information. I'm making risky decisions (for me), like wanting to eat at a restaurant. I love spending money. My brain loses focus easily, forgetting days and tasks. Thoughts skip like a rock on smooth water that eventually must sink and disappear. I deal with medication side effects; excessive sleepiness, high cholesterol, and an insatiable appetite. I weigh far more than my peak pregnancy weight, and purple lines have blossomed up and down my thighs. Things won't go back to normal, but that doesn't matter. I'm home with my baby and with my family.

Holly P is mom to Wyatt and lives in Vancouver, British Columbia. After the birth of her son, she spent two weeks in a psychiatric ward due to postpartum psychosis. Holly plans to return to work as a restaurant manager at the end of her maternity leave. You can find Holly @ postpartumpsychosismom on Instagram.

INTENSE PSYCHOTIC EPISODE

Amanda Scott

PEOPLE HAVE ASKED ME ABOUT my birth story, but I have been too ashamed to share it until now. I have had some time to heal and reflect and at the end of the day, other women sharing their experiences is what got me through. If I can make someone feel less alone and less crazy, then I must share mine, too.

I've learned the hard way that there is very little research on postpartum psychosis and even less on prepartum psychosis (if that's what it's even called). I had the unfortunate experience of suffering from both.

Here goes...

I am pregnant with my third child. My first pregnancy ended in miscarriage at 11.5 weeks. That is where the depression and anxiety started.

This pregnancy is difficult, right from the beginning. I have no energy and a one-year-old to care for. I'm struggling with postpartum depression and anxiety, estrangement from a family member, a rocky relationship with my partner, and finances are a growing concern. My stress levels are at an all-time high.

At 32 weeks pregnant, I receive a call that my grandma, who is a personal hero of mine, is in the hospital and probably won't be with us much longer. This is when the nightmare gets worse.

I'm not getting much sleep to begin with, and now I'm starting to become paranoid and suspicious of my partner. I believe he is having an affair. I pack up my dogs and son at four a.m. and drive two hours to my parents' house. On the way, I stop for coffee and check the baby monitor app on my phone. I hear what I believe to be my husband with another woman, an auditory hallucination. I begin recording everything. I can't put the phone down, and I can't stop listening. I am in absolute shock from what I am hearing. I arrive at my parents' house. They take my son and I head downstairs, glued to my phone.

That same night, or very early morning, I hysterically barge into their bedroom, waking them from their sleep. I am terrified, shaking, and in tears. I tell them that my partner has another girlfriend and they are planning to kill me, that I heard everything on a live stream on my phone. (The live stream doesn't exist.) It is clear as day to me, but my parents say they can't hear anything. I am convinced that my partner and his new lover are spying on all of us and they can see us at this very moment.

I am hearing irrational, crazy, disturbing things that make no sense. I believe my husband and his supposed girlfriend have found out I know about their plot to murder me so now they are talking behind my back to others, trying to destroy my character and take my son from me. I can hear the girlfriend reading my private journals in my home and laughing at me. I think they are hacking into my phone, so I spend hours changing my passwords over and over because every time I change it I think they have already figured it out.

Since no one can hear the voices except me, I begin to believe that maybe I am gifted with hearing things in another frequency that others can't hear, that maybe I am clairaudient.

It feels like torture, and I believe that I can't live like this but that I can't die because my son needs me. I can't leave him alone with his father, now that I know he is a monster and has an evil girlfriend.

Soon, the voices I am hearing on my phone become a constant running commentary. I lock my phone in the trunk of my car, but the voices follow me. I can't escape them. I hear new voices as well, and they're all conspiring against me. I am terrified and desperate to protect my son and unborn child. I call the police and tell them about the plot by my husband his girlfriend to murder me and that I need protection. I call a friend's mom, a previous social worker, for her advice. I call a well-established lawyer I briefly worked with years ago for legal advice and representation. I go to the courthouse to seek an emergency protective order. I send all of the recordings I made on my phone to a forensic sound professional who later confirms there is absolutely nothing audible other than my cat meowing.

I show up at the police station looking for protection. I call a neighbour to watch my house because I think the evil woman, my husband's supposed girlfriend, is hiding in my home. I call the police to have them search my house because I am convinced she is there and I am afraid to leave my parents' and go home. The police offer to escort me home when I'm ready and suggest having my parents come with me.

All of this happens in the span of a week. My family is afraid to take me to the hospital for help because they don't know what is happening, or if there is any truth to what I am saying. They are afraid I will have my children taken away. Meanwhile, my partner is completely unaware that any of this is happening. He is hosting a work retreat at the time.

During this time, I am also hearing hidden messages through the radio. I believe all the songs have a secret meaning. I am insisting that family members turn their phones off and put them in the trunk so we can't be heard or tracked. I think I am being followed. I'm not eating or sleeping. I have poor hygiene. I lose ten pounds in five days, and my pregnancy becomes high risk. I thank God I was with my parents when this all happened. I shudder to think of what could have happened to my son if they weren't there to help care for him.

I am at the hospital with family when my grandma passes. Attempting to act normal, say goodbye, and be there to support my grieving family, I am privately hearing cruel, obscene voices.

The intense psychotic episode lasts a week, though I remain paranoid for months. The anxiety that follows is crippling, but I believe it is very important that I act as normal as possible and shine as a mother. I am still terrified of losing my children. I have zero intention of telling my partner, because I am mortified with my behaviour and afraid of how he will react Weeks later, we receive a visit from a social worker because of one of the phone calls I made during the psychosis. At this point, I have to tell my partner what happened. Although I don't think he will ever fully understand because he didn't witness it, he is incredibly understanding and supportive.

A month later my partner and I welcome a beautiful, healthy baby girl. It's been two and a half years since the psychosis, and it's been a difficult journey rebuilding my confidence. Forgiving myself for what I put my family through and making peace with the unbearable guilt, shame ,and humiliation has been a challenge.

I think it's important to note that I had no previous history of mental illness other than the postpartum depression and anxiety I was struggling with at the time. I later learned that I was completely nutritionally depleted as a result of three consecutive pregnancies. I was also anemic and had thyroid issues.

Amanda Scott is a mom of two and lives in Calgary, Alberta. Her Facebook Page is called PMAD Healing and Recovery and you can also find Amanda on Instagram @pmadhealingandrecovery

MY VILLAGE SAVED ME

Dr. Anita Ewan

AS A CHILD, THE FUTURE I envisioned for myself always included being a mother. What the vision didn't include was me wanting to kill my infant the day I brought her home.

I had my baby at the age of eighteen and moved out of my family home shortly before giving birth. When I came home from the hospital, it was just me and my baby in our large and empty two bedroom townhouse.

Ella, my baby, is crying, and I am unable to comfort her. I feed her and change her diaper, but the crying never stops. I try rocking her to sleep to no avail. Negative voices slowly begin to creep into my mind.

She's better off without you. You'll never be able to keep her alive.

I begin experiencing an odd feeling of peace when I conjure up the idea of smothering my baby with a pillow. I just want her to stop crying, not because her crying annoys me—although it makes me extremely anxious—I only want her to stop suffering. That's what my mind tells me.

I am making my baby suffer. I am an unfit mother.

I pick up the phone and call my aunty. She was the first person I called when I found out I was pregnant and would be a teenage mother. I was unable to tell my strict Christian mother. I feared she would throw me out of the house. My aunty was Christian, too, but she was super supportive. She told me babies are a blessing and assured me that although my mother would be very upset, she would be a loving grandmother. This eased my anxiety and helped me tremendously. Now, once again, she provides me with a similar type of invaluable support.

"Aunty, I can't do this," I say, bawling uncontrollably over the phone.

"You can't do what?" she asks. "Where's the baby?"

"She's right here, in my arms," I reply. "She won't stop crying. I can't make her stop, Aunty. I'm a terrible mother".

My aunty calmly but firmly tells me to take a deep breath and slow down. She then asks me if I've fed the baby.

"Yes," I answer.

"Is your baby's diaper dry?" she asks.

"Yes," I reply.

My aunty reassures me that my baby is safe and that sometimes they cry because of reasons we don't immediately know at first. If the baby is fed and clean, then she is okay for the most part.

The next question she asks, saves my life and that of my baby's.

"When was the last time *you* slept?"

I stop and realize that I haven't slept since I came home from the hospital earlier that day. I tell my aunty this.

"Anita, you need sleep," she says. "Put the baby down and go lie down. Make sure your baby is warm and go rest. Your baby will be okay. You need to make sure you sleep so you don't lose your mind."

Turns out my sweet baby Ella is cold and tired. She is unable to sleep because she isn't wearing enough layers and I did not wrap her properly. I follow aunty's instructions, retrieve a long onesie and a blanket to make sure Ella is warm enough, and she falls right to sleep.

Once Ella stops crying, I realize how exhausted I am. Before hanging up with my aunty, she reminds me to eat and makes me promise I will go and rest. After putting Ella into her bassinet, I go downstairs and eat a small snack and go right to sleep.

Both Ella and I sleep through the night. I am awakened by a phone call. It's my mother. My aunty called her to tell her what had happened. She says she is coming over, and a couple hours later she arrives. She decides to stay for a few weeks to help me transition into motherhood. Five children in, and she has done this for each one of my postpartum recoveries.

It's hard for me to think back to the night I was having challenges with my daughter. And it's even harder to think about what would have happened if I did not have my aunty to reach out to during that time. But it's important for me to reflect on that night and share my story to provide the realities of postpartum psychosis and how dangerous it can be if left untreated.

I also wanted to highlight the lack of resources some mothers have during this time. I know particularly as a Black teenage mother, I was uncomfortable calling the police or emergency services to help me through the negative thoughts. I knew that children's services would be involved, an organization I distrust. I would have rather died (or at the time, killed my baby) than have my baby torn away from me and be stripped of my maternal rights.

I now wonder what it would have been like if there was an organization I trusted to reach out to when I was in distress. How great and reassuring would it have been to have someone come and stay with me and help me get through the rest of the night.

I thank God each day for my aunty and mommy. They say it takes a village to raise a child, it also took one to save our lives.

Dr. Anita Ewan is a mom of five and lives in Toronto, Ontario. She is a child development specialist and teaches at three universities and is also an ethnographer and research consultant with the Government of Canada.

WE DESERVE BETTER

Renae Real

THE DAY I WAS DISCHARGED from the hospital after giving birth was the day my mom and husband noticed something wasn't right. I was talking a mile a minute. I hadn't been able to sleep much in the hospital. I felt like I had boundless energy and my thoughts were racing like crazy.

I agreed to have them call a public health nurse to come to the house the next day.

They sent a woman from the psychiatric ward instead. I told her that I was terrified that I would be separated from my son, and she promised me that that would not happen. She set up an appointment for me to see a doctor at the hospital for later that day.

A few hours before my scheduled appointment, I was in a total delirium. My mom stayed with the baby, and my husband rushed me to the hospital. From there, they told him I had to be admitted to the psychiatric ward. I remember my husband leaving, and I was wheeled away. This is when our nightmare started.

Four days after giving birth to my first child, I found myself committed to our local hospital under the Mental Health Act.

I was diagnosed with postpartum psychosis, but I was not made aware of my diagnosis until my husband explained it on one of his visits. I believed I had suffered a psychotic break from exhaustion. I blamed myself for ending up in the psychiatric ward and felt so much shame and guilt. I had no idea that birth trauma, exhaustion, and hormones contributed to my illness, or that I had an actual diagnosable condition, that was rare but not unique.

I was scared I would never be myself again. I was confused and felt desperately alone.

I was held in hospital against my will. Every day, I asked to go home. I was isolated from the other patients and only allowed one short visit from my husband and son per day. My requests to see a counsellor, seek spiritual guidance, and to talk to a social worker were all denied. I was not allowed outside for fresh air, and I could not mingle with the other patients. I had limited access to a phone and zero information. The other patients had rights I did not have, and I felt that I was being punished. When I asked to know my rights, the charge nurse told me I had none.

I wanted to have the facts. I needed to understand what had happened to me—seemingly overnight. The lack of information and isolation drove me to the brink of insanity. I was afraid that they would never let me out.

I had approximately 45 minutes with the psychiatrist on staff over my 17-day stay. He never explained my condition. For close to three weeks, he cancelled meetings with me to prioritize other patients. The psychiatrist tried to discourage me from pumping my breast milk, implying that it was *too much for me*. I did not feel heard or valued. He was more interested in sharing his professional accomplishments and anecdotes about his wife's experience with bottle feeding rather than hearing the issues unique to me and my care. Breastfeeding was and continues to be an incredibly important part of my journey. If it weren't for an incredible family doctor who agreed to take on my care, visiting me almost daily, I would have lost complete hope.

When I pressed staff for more information, I was told to settle down, not to worry, and not to get too emotional. It felt like I was in a 1950s horror movie and about to be diagnosed with a wandering uterus. It felt like I had landed myself in the madhouse and had my baby taken from me. The lack of power, authority, and autonomy over my body and medical care left me feeling vulnerable and powerless.

The evening I was admitted, I was put into an isolation room overnight. My glasses were taken from me for my safety, and I was shown to a cot on the floor. A loud door closed behind me, and I was told to go to sleep, despite the intense overhead fluorescent lights that were left on all night.

I was terrified and reliving my delivery but believed that I was delivering a god baby who would grow into an oak tree and save the world from COVID-19 and natural disasters. I couldn't see without my glasses and had to make out my surroundings through touch.

What I discovered was akin to a prison cell.

I was leaking breast milk and was cold and confused. I could not make sense of what was happening to me.

Was I in jail? Was I being tortured? Where was my family? What did I do wrong to deserve this?

My thoughts were racing and my head felt like exploding. The masks the nurses and guards were wearing terrified me. They looked like faceless monsters. I screamed for my family and begged to be let out. I couldn't see, and they were talking to me over a loudspeaker. I started to believe that god was talking to me and punishing me. I pleaded and begged for them to open the door. I was trapped in a concrete cell. There was a steel toilet, a mat on the ground, no sheets, and a thin blanket.

I scurried on the rough concrete floor on my hands and knees feeling the perimeter of the room until I found the door. I put my fingers against the bottom and sobbed while I asked them to open it. In the morning, my legs were covered in scratches and bruises from trying to find a way to escape.

I tried flooding the room using the sink over the toilet, believing they would never leave me in a wet cell. That didn't work. My mind told me to create a raft and sail away. I took the plastic pillow off the cot and kneeled on it. I used my hands to float myself over the wet floor and out the door. Of course, I couldn't sail my way out.

When that didn't work, I believed the pillow had a secret message stashed inside that I could use to escape. I tried to tear it open with my teeth.

None of this worked. I could not escape or will myself out of the situation, no matter how magical and powerful I believed I was.

They would come check on me, but only to order me onto the mat. Telling me to lay still and sleep, which was impossible. I truly believed that I was in labour (again), delivering my god baby, Odin. I couldn't understand why no one wanted to help me bring this baby into the world and why I had to suffer alone. I started to believe that I had to sacrifice my life to bring my god baby into the world. I wanted someone to hold my hand while I delivered my child. With each passing hour I became more and more weak; this was exhaustion setting in but in my mind it was my life leaving my body. My screams turned to quiet sobs.

I could hear the guards and nurses come and go. I could hear them pace the hall, ignoring my pleas. I started to believe it was my family. Leaving me to die because I wasn't worthy of saving.

The delusions grew darker and darker with each passing hour.

The next day my throat ached from screaming, I was covered in dried breast milk and lochia. It was humiliating, dehumanizing, and it felt incredibly shameful. I willed myself to disappear.

They lost my glasses for three days. This was a terrifying experience and it extended my delirium. Despite asking for my glasses continuousl,y no one seemed in a rush to find them.

When I became lucid, I asked why I was held in cells like this. I was told because it was because I was admitted on a Friday and there were no psychiatrists on staff until Monday. I was told it was for my safety and to keep me from disrupting the other patients. The emotional anguish of being left in these conditions continues to haunt me.

I was nervous about having my first child and sought out midwifery care in the neighbouring city. I did everything in my power to have a natural delivery fearing a caesarean section. The idea of being numbed terrified me.

In the end, I avoided drugs (except for laughing gas) and a caesarean delivery, but my son was stuck and was delivered via forceps. I sustained fourth degree tears and required a spinal and 2.5 hours in an operating room to repair the damage. This is when I began to disassociate. I could not handle being away from my husband, away from my brand-new baby, and numb with my legs in stirrups. I was exhausted and felt so vulnerable. It was every one of my fears come true; until I was committed to the psych ward, at least.

I spent 17 excruciating days away from my newborn and my family. I was released with no psychiatric follow-up care except for one appointment with the same psychiatrist one month later, despite asking to be referred to BC Women's Reproductive and Mental Health Program.

Upon my release, my midwife referred me to the program. This is where I believe I should have been referred to on day one, but no one at the hospital bothered to look into more suitable care for me.

When I got home, I was a shell of myself. I have since been diagnosed with post-traumatic stress disorder from the experience and struggle with thoughts of suicide.

Each day, I claw to the surface and decide to fight.

This experience has forever changed me. I share this story despite a deep sense of shame and stigma to highlight the disgraceful state of our perinatal mental health system.

A mother and baby unit (Canada has none) and staff trained to treat perinatal mental health conditions would have made all the difference in my care. It would have spared me the separation from my son, the humiliation I felt and the constant fear I had while being committed with male patients.

I will not stop telling my story until every birthing Canadian has access to the perinatal mental health care we so desperately deserve.

This condition is scary, confusing, and to be frank, complete torture, but the worst part of the ordeal was being separated from my newborn for nearly three weeks while I received care

I had no idea this disease existed or how it would impact my life, but what surprised me the most was the lack of resources for women in Canada.

The pain of the separation leaves deep scars on my heart that I am not sure will ever heal.

We cannot continue to treat mothers and babies his way. It's barbaric.

We deserve better.

Renae Real is mom to Leland and lives in British Columbia. She can be found on Facebook or at renae.real@gmail.com

POSTPARTUM PSYCHOSIS

Dr. Anja Wittkowski

MOST WOMEN MAY HAVE HEARD about the baby blues or even postnatal depression, but the same cannot be said about postpartum psychosis. Postpartum psychosis, which has also been referred to as puerperal psychosis or psychosis after childbirth, describes a psychotic episode that women experience within the first two weeks after childbirth, with symptoms typically beginning by day three after birth or even during labour1. However, women seem to be less at risk of developing it after the first three months after childbirth.

As its incidence can range from 0.89 to 2.6 in 1000 women, which translates into 1 to 2 new mothers being affected, it is a rare condition, especially when compared to postnatal depression with a prevalence of 4%-63.9% globally. However, it is important to recognize that the relative risk for a first onset of postpartum psychosis is 23 times higher within four weeks following childbirth compared with any other period during a woman's life. Thus, postpartum psychosis is a severe and acute psychiatric disorder, if not the most severe disorder associated with childbirth. It is classed as a medical emergency, often requiring admission to a psychiatric hospital and ideally a Mother and Baby Unit (MBU), if one exists in the region or country. As the mental health of women affected tends to deteriorate so quickly, women should be assessed by a mental health team within four hours. The diagnosis is normally made by a psychiatrist.

What are the symptoms of postpartum psychosis?

If women search the Internet using the term postpartum psychosis, they may come across a list of symptoms that include:

- hallucinations—hearing voices or seeing things
- delusions—thoughts or beliefs that are unlikely to be true

- manic mood—talking and thinking too much or too quickly, feeling "high" or "on top of the world" or loosing inhibitions
- low mood—showing signs of depression, being withdrawn or tearful, lacking energy, having a loss of appetite, anxiety or trouble sleeping
- feeling suspicious, fearful, restless or very confused
- behaving in a way that's out of character

Symptoms of postpartum psychosis include hallucinations and delusional beliefs, which are often coupled with changes in mood so that women may also experience symptoms of mania including elation, excess energy, racing thoughts and restlessness or symptoms of depression including beliefs and feelings of helplessness, hopelessness and worthlessness or indeed both. Women may express delusional beliefs that often focus on childbirth or obsessive thoughts about their baby. Women may think that their baby is in danger, for example, of being stolen or hurt, but they may also believe that their baby is an evil spirit or the devil. They may show disorganised, unusual behaviours and appear disorientated and confused8. As women may not realize that they are experiencing a severe mental illness, the UK National Health Service (NHS) website warns women to "be aware that if you have postpartum psychosis, you may not realise you're ill. Your partner, family or friends may spot the signs and have to take action."

These symptoms or experiences may sound scary, and in some cases they can have significant impacts, such as an involuntary admission to hospital and women not being able to care appropriately for their baby during this time. In the worst of cases, postpartum psychosis can result in extremely tragic outcomes including the mother's death by suicide or the mother posing a threat to the baby's life; however, it should be stressed that only 19% of 130 women admitted to a MBU experienced suicidal thoughts and only 8% experienced thoughts about killing their baby11. Whilst not all women who experience postpartum psychosis contemplate taking their own lives during the course of this illness, it is undeniable that these symptoms cause considerable distress to the women and can initially impact the bond developing between the mother and her baby. However, women with postpartum psychosis recover relatively rapidly, within a few weeks, and this means they can resume caring for their baby quickly.

What factors may make it more likely for postpartum psychosis to develop?

There may be certain factors that increase a woman's risk to develop postpartum psychosis, such as being a first-time mother. Other examined risk factors include younger age, lower income, perinatal and neonatal complications and a past hospitalization for psychiatric disorder. Stress may also be implicated. Women are also at increased risk if they or family members have had a previous episode or have bipolar disorder[1]. Thus, both biological and environmental factors may be implicated in increasing a woman's risk to develop this condition. However, for many women, it is difficult to identify any specific factors that may have predisposed them.

What is the prognosis?

Whilst postpartum psychosis can impair a woman's insight into her wellbeing, the overall prognosis or outlook in terms of recovery is good. For example, most mothers with postpartum psychosis tend to be discharged within the average duration of a MBU admission of seven weeks. In addition, the majority of women, who required inpatient treatment, reported to have recovered when asked nine months after giving birth: with 88% having resumed their work and home responsibilities. Thus, the prognosis is excellent, including women's psychological recovery. However, preconception counselling is advisable for those mothers considering having another child[1].

How is postpartum psychosis treated?

Treatment normally involves admission to hospital and specifically to an inpatient, psychiatric unit or a MBU so that mother and baby can stay together[1]. For example, the UK NICE[1] guidelines (evidence-based recommendations for health care in England) advise that these mothers should receive specialist treatment through a MBU admission and its multidisciplinary team of psychiatric staff, nursery nurses and clinical psychologists. Admission to a MBU has been found to improve the mother's mental health, the mother-infant relationship and child development30. In a study of 25 mothers and their babies admitted to an Australian MBU, researchers noted that 64% were admitted involuntarily; all mothers were treated with antipsychotic medication and 36% were able to continue breastfeeding. The babies of these mothers were observed to have developed normally during the admission. all mothers were discharged with their infants in their care.

However, MBUs do not exist in every country, meaning that treatment options will vary and, as a psychiatric emergency, medication plays a major role in treatment1. Treatment with antipsychotic medication alone or in combination with other psychiatric medications leads to faster mental health improvements and a quicker discharge from hospital32. However, any medication and intervention should be tailored to the woman, her symptoms and needs.

Postpartum psychosis is a severe perinatal mental illness, but it is rare and, importantly, women tend to improve quickly with treatment and recover well.

Dr. Anja Wittkowski is a senior lecturer/associate professor in clinical psychology in the Division of Psychology and Mental Health, School of Health Sciences, at The University of Manchester. She is also working as a Health and Care Professions Council registered clinical psychologist for the Greater Manchester Mental Health NHS Foundation Trust (GMMH). As the lead of GMMH's Perinatal Mental Health and Parenting Research Unit (PRIME-RU), Dr Wittkowski specializes in perinatal clinical psychology and the primary aim of her research is to trial psychological and parenting interventions to enhance parental wellbeing and the parent-infant-relationship and modify family risk factors. For example, she was the Manchester Lead and co-applicant for the National Institute Health Research (NIHR) Public Health Research funded THRIVE trial (Henderson, Wittkowski, et al. 2013-2019) and the Principal Investigator for the NIHR Research for Patient Benefit funded feasibility trial of the Baby Triple P Positive Parenting Programme for mothers with severe mental heatlh difficulties, called the IMAgINE study (Wittkowski et al., 2016-2019).

Part 5:

A Pandemic
&
the Future
of Mental Health

patience
a quality all mothers possess
it starts in the womb
learned from awaiting our baby's arrival

Tyneisha Ternent @tythepoetess

SWEET BABY ADA

Candice Thomas

My sweet baby Ada...

This year was nothing like we had planned. Being pregnant was hard enough without having to live through an unprecedented pandemic.

Now you are here. And the pandemic shows no signs of slowing down.

We are in lockdown.

Again.

In the middle of winter.

And it's just so damn hard.

Oh Ada, how I wish your first visitor at the hospital could have been your sister. From four floors down, she saw you through the window, and I know she loved you all the same.

But it's still hard.

I wish my mom got to hold you when you were only hours old.

I wish you could get to see my dad more before he forgets who you are. His memory might hold him back, but the smile you bring to his face is priceless. He sees you for the first time, every time, and that's special.

I wish you could meet your cousins. You'd love them. They are just as wild and free as your sister.

I wish I wasn't so tired.

I have found my anxiety and depression slowly increasing since the pandemic started. Since I shut down my business and became a stay at home, working mom, it all feels so overwhelming with no end in sight.

COVID-19 has changed the way I cope because often going out to visit family and friends was part of my routine to decompress. Now, even though I can see them virtually, it is not the same. The connection just isn't the same.

I've had days where I don't get out of bed. I cry for a few hours, and sometimes just putting my coat on to go outside for a walk seems like too much for me. I have to be strong for my daughters, but as the days go by, it's getting harder and harder.

Sometimes people will say "You can do it, it'll pass," but that just makes me feel like I'm in a world of my own, like they don't see or feel what I'm feeling, like a car is running me over but they don't see the car, they just see me lying down and want me to just get up.

As if it's that easy. I so wish it were.

My anxiety grows. It keeps me up at night. Suffering from perinatal mental illness during a pandemic is a literal nightmare. Most days feel impossible to get through.

Most days I just want to stay asleep.

It's lonely but I have a newborn and a toddler to care for.

It's so hard.

The crying never stops. The sleepless nights never end. How could this be happening to me? I was not ready for any of this. Why didn't anyone tell me it would be this challenging?

I can't handle the "witching hour" or, in my case, the hours. I sit outside on my front steps even though it is the middle of winter and freezing. I close my eyes and take four or five deep breaths, hoping that will help.

When I look down the street I keep thinking, *I want to run away. I want to be like the people I see walking by. They are free and I'm not. I feel like there is an invisible chain holding me to this small human that won't stop crying.*

I instantly feel guilty for thinking these things, but I feel them so deeply. I cannot escape the thoughts. I can hear you crying, Ada. I know I have to go back inside. I tell myself, *You can do this,* as tears run down my face. I walk back into the house, and my husband hands me a screaming helpless baby I hardly know.

They say it is love at first sight, but how do you love someone you've never met? I never got that feeling of deep connection right away. Is there something wrong with me? Did I do something wrong? Maybe I am just not a good mom and this baby can feel it.

It's lonely at night and always so dark, and I know the darkest days and nights are coming. I do not have the energy to speak to anyone, but when I do, I feel like they are not listening. I tell them, "I am lonely; I cannot do this; I'm exhausted." But the response is always the same: "I know it must be hard but you are strong; you will get through it." Why can't anyone just sit with me and be a presence instead of an opinion? If my mother-in-law tells me one more time: "Well, we didn't do it like that in my day," I might just snap. I'm doing the best I can.

The sadness is all consuming. The anxiety makes me feel like I am constantly drowsy and gasping for air. I don't know if this is a battle I can win. I feel like giving up, but I am scared to leave my baby. She needs me. Thoughts of not being here anymore creep up, and some days I don't have the energy to fight them.

I am terrified.

Who can help me?

Candice Thomas is a mom of two and lives in Barrie, Ontario. She is a registered massage therapist and creates online mindfulness-based programs for help with anxiety and depression. You can find Candice on Instagram @evergreen_rmt and @livmohrproject

I THINK I NEED HELP

Laura Stinnett

FROM DAY ONE OF BEING pregnant with my second daughter, Taylor, I was sick as a dog until about 17 weeks. I was working full time at a very high stress job with a two-year-old at home. There weren't many chances to nap or lie down and watch TV when I wasn't feeling well. I started to feel a little better around the holidays and thought maybe everything would be fine and normal.

Then COVID-19 hit, and that's when the shit really hit the fan.

I was in my third trimester, way fucking bigger than I'd ever been in my life and way fucking nervous about this global pandemic. How was I going to keep my unborn child and three-year-old safe and healthy?

I had to start working from home because of the pandemic. So now I was about 8.5 months pregnant working from home with a toddler. I was stressed.

Since my first was a C-section baby, I opted for another one this time around due to my ever-increasing anxiety. I needed to have some control over what was going to happen.

Well, as we moms know, most things with kids don't go according to plan.

I went into labor days before I was scheduled to go in for my induction. Taylor Madison was born, and she was the sweetest, chubbiest thing ever.

Because of COVID, it was just the three of us for a few days in the hospital—the baby, me, and my husband.

After days of trouble breastfeeding and of course not sleeping, I began to spiral. On the day we were supposed to go home, I started to feel a lot of anxiety, very much like I did after my first when I suffered from postpartum anxiety.

I thought to myself, *Crap, here we go.* My husband left the hospital that morning to go home, shower, and get my toddler so she could meet her baby sister for the first time. It wasn't a meeting like I had dreamed because of stupid COVID. She couldn't come see us in the hospital so we had to meet her in the car. She was out of sorts and tired but stared at her new little sister the entire way home.

I felt relieved to be home, but six days later, after crying the whole time we were home, I hit my breaking point. I looked at my husband and muttered, "I think I need help." The look on his face was a look of familiarity and terror at the same time.

I felt like my husband and the girls would be better off without me. I was so embarrassed that those thoughts would even enter my mind and felt so sorry that my husband and sweet girls had this loser for a wife and mom.

I called my aunt, someone I felt comfortable with, and told her. She suggested I call my obstetrician immediately. I did, but the after-hours, answering service picked up. I am a blubbering mess, trying to explain to the woman on the phone that I need to speak with the on-call doctor because I am having some kind of perinatal mental health episode. She then told me that she couldn't prescribe any medication but that sometimes when you get the baby blues, going for a nice walk or taking a bath helps.

Thankfully, I do finally get to speak with a doctor and receive a script for anti-anxiety medication.

This time around, the postpartum anxiety hit me hard and fast. It was dark. I wonder if it's because I was way more stressed the second time, you know, being right in the middle of a global pandemic and all and trying to parent without ever getting a break.

At my follow- up appointment with the midwife, she tells me to work on getting at least six hours of sleep a night, eat whole nutrient-rich food, drink tons of water, get outside, move my body, and start seeing a therapist. Easier said than done but I had a lot of help around me to get it all done.

I am five months postpartum now and starting to feel better. But now we're in wave two of this never-ending raging pandemic and the anxiety is returning.

Crap, here we go again.

Laura Stinett is a mom of two and lives in Denver, Colorado. Laura has a blog lameredotblog.wordpress.com and you can find her on Instagram @Bof2queens

LOCKDOWN

Lindsay Gareau

Our family of four has become a family of five with the birth of our youngest daughter, Charlotte. My eldest daughters, Elena, five, and Chloe, two and a half, are thrilled to have another little sister to play with and dote over.

The first six weeks fly by and are as normal as normal can be during the ups and down and sleepless nights of the newborn phase.

But then we start hearing about a virus affecting different parts of the world.

There are just a few infections here, and any concerns regarding what they are now calling the COVID-19 virus does not yet rank high on my list of worries. Interactions with friends and family continue as planned, along with various scheduled events such as Charlotte's upcoming baby shower.

Within a few days of the baby shower, Saskatchewan suddenly declares a state of emergency, schools are closed indefinitely, and because our daycare is attached to a school. This means, not only do I have my colicky newborn to deal with at home, I now suddenly also have my two eldest children to entertain.

I did not sign up for this. Parenting in a pandemic is hard, of that there is no doubt.

This year should have been an amazing year filled with love, laughter, family, and play dates. I console myself by believing these measures are only temporary. A week later, all non-essential businesses are closed and gatherings are limited to ten people.

Now I'm beginning to worry. We decide not to gather with extended family so as not to expose ourselves to this rapidly spreading virus. We try to adapt to our new normal and I am still able to get support from family.

What comes next is absolutely devastating.

The government mandates contact be limited to household members only.

We are now in full lockdown. I am in shock.

As a mom with three kids under five, I think, *How can I do this?* The week prior, I saw my parents daily and had lunch dates with friends. I am sad and mad and frustrated and scared.

Society tells us that it takes a village to raise a child, but the lockdown has taken away my village. How is this going to work? It's okay. "It's just temporary" is a phrase that becomes my daily mantra, but as time goes on, the situation just gets worse.

More restrictions. Now, not only are we limited to seeing people only within our own household, we are told that shopping is only for essential items and outdoor parks will close. The city places caution tape on all play structures.

The conversation on social media starts off positive. I see a lot of messages like "*ca va aller*" (It will be alright) and "we're in this together." A temporary reset is how I choose to view these extreme measures.

I am also hopeful they will force us to slow down, enjoy more quality time with our families, and even help us be more loving and understanding towards one another. But unfortunately the opposite starts happening. I start to see people becoming critical of one another and judgmental of other's choices (i.e. toilet paper hoarding, choosing certain family bubbles over others, etc.).

I am out grocery shopping with my infant when it starts pouring. An employee walks out with me and uses an umbrella to shield my infant. While I get the baby into the car, this kind young man holds the umbrella over me as I load the groceries in. I thank him for his help, and he returns to the store. That's when I realize I still have the shopping cart to put away a little distance from the car, but I can't leave my baby unattended. I ask a passing stranger if she would kindly mind taking the cart to the cart holder to the store for me, but she turns to me and states harshly that if I can't handle shopping with a baby during a pandemic, then maybe I shouldn't be here at all.

Instead of becoming angry and upset, it's in this moment I make the decision to practice more kindness with others and to teach my daughters how powerful our behaviour and words can be to others around us.

Spring is here and it's time to celebrate because after a long winter lockdown, we are now allowed to expand our bubbles. Little do I know that the new changes to our province's easing of pandemic restrictions would be equally as hard as when the lockdown came into force.

Our family is presented with a choice of choosing who to include into our new inner circle. This sounds easy in theory, however, considering unique family dynamics and personalities, this task proves to be quite difficult.

As an only child, it is easy to make the decision to include my parents into our inner circle. Incorporating my in-laws into our bubble, however, is less than straightforward. My husband has three siblings here in Regina where we live, two of which have kids close in age to mine. This means some family members would need to be chosen over others.

From this moment on, every single decision we make has to be carefully thought out as every choice is scrutinized and criticized by family members. This new pandemic obstacle is challenging my natural people-pleasing tendencies, but I need to make decisions that are best for my core family, trusting that others are doing the same. This is causing some hurt feelings due to the difficult decisions that have to be made, and we are still attempting to mend these relationships months later.

Not only is this hard on us adults who theoretically understand the situation, but trying to explain our decisions to our children is exceptionally challenging. My eldest daughter really struggles not being able to see her grandparents, cousins, and best friend on a regular basis. I try to explain the reason for the disruption to her routine and why are restricting her social interactions by telling her it is only temporary and that we're doing it to keep people safe.

She is angry and lashes out at me for these limitations. She is missing her people and I am missing mine, so together we find ways of trying to connect with our loved ones daily through FaceTime calls and with drive-by visits where we remain in the car.

I hate that we can't hug our family and friends for now. I am huge on hugs. It's how we raise our girls, telling them that hugs can help fix anything. Our conversations with our girls often include brainstorming sessions on finding different ways to express our love and appreciation for others.

How can we show love and receive love that's not through physical touch? I need to figure this out for me, for my girls, so that they don't grow up fearing physical touch or missing a crucial part of connection. We begin filling out a gratitude book daily to help us see the good in our day-to-day interactions. This is something positive that I hope my daughters will take from this strange time.

As a family, we have had to learn how to combat forced isolation and unforeseen hardships in very creative ways. We have learned to use the technology that has been distancing us from others to connect. We have learned to improve our communication of feelings with each other, even when it hurts. We have learned to support our local businesses and actively practice expressing kindness in our daily lives.

As I reflect over the events of the last year and my maternity leave ending soon, I find myself releasing any anger or frustration I may have carried with me over these trying months. I have found a new sense of gratitude. I am grateful for my family. My baby is going to turn one, my children are healthy, and my husband has been fortunate enough to keep his job. We have found ways to show gratitude and love to others through non-traditional means, Zoom game nights, car parades for birthday celebrations, and socially distanced garage visits. Although this past year has been challenging in so many ways, I am blessed. I am thankful we are all well and healthy and most of all, that we made it through a year that we never imagined would be a reality.

Lindsay Gareau is a mom of three and lives in Regina, Saskatchewan. She has a master of social work and counsels moms with perinatal mood and anxiety disorders. Lindsay's Facebook Page is called Prairie Heart Counselling Inc.

VIRTUAL CARE

Dr. Ariel Dalfen

PRIOR TO THE COVID-19 PANDEMIC, the mental health care system in Canada was already overburdened and unable to meet the needs of many Canadians. COVID-19 seems to have led to increasing rates of psychiatric distress, illness, and devastating outcomes. The mental health impacts of COVID will likely linger for Canadians for many years to come. This is particularly true in the perinatal population where women have struggled with anxiety and fear about getting COVID while pregnant, during delivery in the hospital, or as the mother of a newborn, being isolated at home as a new parent and being cut-off from regular support people and programs, and are facing the significant financial and health concerns alongside other Canadians.

Since the onset of COVID-19, virtual medical care has become increasingly acceptable and widespread, but this was not always the case. For many years, my colleagues and I at Mount Sinai Hospital in Toronto were unique in delivering psychiatric care via telemedicine to women all over Ontario, in order for them to get the type of specialized mental health care they need.

Even though effective treatments exist, only 20% of affected women suffering from perinatal mental health disorders receive sufficient care. Barriers to the access and uptake of treatment include stigma, fear of child protective services being called, and confusion about what are "normal" feelings for a new mother to experience versus symptoms of a psychiatric illness. Additionally, there are financial and logistical barriers that limit attendance at an appointment, such as lack of time, limited childcare, scheduling and transportation issues, since most treatment centers are located in downtown areas of major Canadian cities. It is also often challenging for women struggling with mobility restrictions or major mental health symptoms during pregnancy or postpartum to travel long distances.

In the field of perinatal mental health care, we have been grappling with these obstacles for many years. Improving access to mental health care, and making it more "user friendly" at this crucial life stage, have been the foci of much of my 15 year career as a perinatal psychiatrist. I have tried to develop and implement virtual care treatment options so that women and their families can more easily find the type of care they need, and access it, regardless of where they live.

Virtual care is defined as "any interaction, whether synchronous or asynchronous in nature between patients and/or members of their circle of care, without direct in person contact, using any form of communication or information technology." (Digital Health Canada, November 2019) Virtual connections in health care can be made using various modalities and technologies, including interactive video meetings on computers or mobile devices, telephone calls, or text messages. These are accessible and familiar technologies that most Canadians already rely on personally and professionally.

The Mount Sinai Hospital Perinatal Mental Health Program is a specialized program that offers psychiatric care to women grappling with mental health issues as they plan pregnancy, during pregnancy and up to one year postpartum. I have been the head of this program since 2009. In 2014, our team created a telemedicine program to address some of the barriers to psychiatric care in this vulnerable population around Ontario.

It took over one year to create this program at that time, and multiple privacy, legal, and other systemic barriers had to be addressed and tackled. To my knowledge, this is the first specific telemedicine program to address the needs of the perinatal population. Through our telemedicine program, women can be seen for psychiatric assessment around medication and treatment planning during pregnancy, while nursing, and during the first year postpartum.

Originally, telemedicine by real-time video consultation was used to connect with women in remote areas of the province who could not otherwise access specialized psychiatric care. In 2014, physicians in our telemedicine program saw 46 new patients, and completed 186 video appointments. Over the years, and with significant investment in change management and education for providers, all of our mental health care providers were trained to use telemedicine, and slowly adapted to providing care, for women when required and when appropriate. Patients reported high rates of satisfaction with this clinical service and enjoyed significant financial and time savings, and did not need to take time off work or find child care to attend an appointment.

As a result, our team's use of telemedicine grew. We used it routinely, throughout the day, and alternated between video and in-person visits, depending on the needs and barriers of a given patient. Decisions to use video visits were made jointly between patients and their mental health care providers. In 2019, our clinicians provided about 200 new patient consultations via telemedicine and over 1400 video appointments to patients around Ontario.

When the COVID-19 pandemic shocked Canada in mid-March 2020, and in-person hospital visits were limited, our team was well positioned to transition to near fully virtual care. New patient assessments, as well as individual and group therapies rapidly transitioned to being virtual, within days.

Between March and July of 2020, approximately 250 new patient consults were done via telemedicine and there were over 2150 video appointments completed by mental health care providers, including psychiatrists, social workers and nursing staff. Group therapies were also quickly converted to virtual care. Enrollment for these groups increased from about 15 participants pre-COVID, to approximately 30 participants on virtual platforms.

Overall, both patients and health care providers have found that using telemedicine has been a positive experience and has enabled vital mental health care to exist when none might be available otherwise. This was true for the perinatal population well before the pandemic limited in person care, and has been particularly striking during COVID. As health care providers, we feel honoured and proud that patients around Ontario invite us into their homes and share their difficult experiences with us. We are proud that we have created a way to offer our services to women in all corners of Ontario and that many women and their families did not experience disruptions in their care due to the pandemic, and that technology can assist us in connecting with pregnant women and new mothers who have been experiencing an increased burden of mental health issues during the pandemic.

It is vital that we continue to be able to reach new mothers and their families in their own homes, in order to be able to provide the psychiatric care that is now more important than ever. It is also essential that we continue to develop virtual care treatment options that do not further accentuate the disparities in accessing mental health care and continue to understand which patients cannot access virtual care and how to improve outreach. My hope for pregnant women and new mothers is that the COVID virtual care boom enables more women to access various types of care, from psychotherapies to psychiatric care, and to obtain effective mental health care, regardless of where they live or socio-economic factors. Systemic issues, such as improving Internet service around the province, funding psychotherapies, funding innovation and the creation, development and evaluation of virtual care treatment options, and the training and compensation of mental health care providers will all be additional considerations to developing and sustaining a vibrant virtual mental health care system well beyond COVID. Fortunately, many of these seeds have been planted and mental health care providers and patients are unlikely to return to pre-COVID levels of in-person mental health care. I look forward to being a part of a future where women and their families can overcome traditional barriers to care and can access an array of treatment options that will help them thrive as parents and as people.

Dr. Ariel Dalfen is Head, Perinatal Mental Health Program and Head, Perinatal Mental Health Telemedicine Program at Mount Sinai Hospital and an Assistant Professor, Psychiatry, University of Toronto. Her research focuses on the use of modern technologies and community collaboration to improve access to care for women with perinatal mental health concerns. Connect with Dr. Dalfen on Twitter @akdalfen

NAVIGATING THE SYSTEM

Tanya Nayler

THE PANDEMIC CHANGED LIFE AS we knew it. I was pregnant and trying to work full-time from home while caring for a preschooler and worried the whole time about the prospect of giving birth without my husband present or worse, contracting COVID-19 at the hospital. Because of my history of anxiety and depression and the significant life stress I was experiencing, I knew I was at risk of postpartum depression. I asked my obstetrician for a referral to the regional perinatal mental health program.

While I waited for a call from the program and my baby's arrival, I decided to speak up about the pandemic's impacts on new and expectant mothers. Suddenly the villages we're told to rely on were no longer available. I wrote an op-ed for a local publication and letters to provincial and federal politicians about the need for more support. I urged my member of parliament, a sitting cabinet minister, to heed the call for a national perinatal mental health strategy. Her office never responded.

When I gave birth, the experience at the hospital was vastly different than the first time I had given birth. I had to check into the hospital alone during active labour, and wore a mask until I started throwing up. My husband was able to join me once I was in a room, but I never got to see the smile behind his mask when our son was born. After delivery, we were confined to a shared room, and the longer we stayed the more I worried about possible exposure to COVID-19.

I was happy to get home as soon as possible afterwards, but I quickly became overwhelmed. At my six-week postpartum follow-up, I mentioned to my obstetrician I hadn't heard yet from the perinatal mental health program. She said because of high demand it could be a long wait, but she would send an updated referral.

While I continued to wait for a call from the program, we entered the highest risk age period for sudden infant death syndrome (SIDS). I was deeply afraid my son would die of SIDS, and despite using a device that monitored his oxygen and heart rate, I still had trouble sleeping. My fear started snowballing, and I started obsessively checking not just my newborn's breathing, but my three-year-old's as well. I also became deeply afraid of losing my children for other reasons. If I heard a noise in the middle of the night, often a wandering cat, I would worry someone had kidnapped one of my boys in their sleep. I became suspicious of people who smiled at my kids or who stopped at the community mailbox across the street from our house. Public health messaging to stay home, although necessary, fueled my anxiety. Anytime I needed to run an errand, I worried about potentially exposing my family, and my newborn, to a deadly virus and whether I could live with myself if the worst happened.

As my exhaustion increased and my anxiety worsened, I made an appointment with my family doctor to talk about my mental health. I was afraid if I disclosed how much I was struggling, I might be involuntarily admitted and separated from my nursing infant. Fortunately, I was not at that point and my doctor referred me to a guided self-help program for anxiety and depression. Although the program's website suggested I would hear from someone within five days, it took about two months to receive an initial call to schedule an intake appointment a month later. Two days before the appointment, I received the tragic news my brother had died of a suspected drug overdose.

My brother and I were less than a year apart in age, and we were like twins growing up. In his twenties, he developed bipolar disorder and substance use disorder, but we remained close. I tried to support him the best I could. After the birth of my second son, I became so overwhelmed with my own struggles, I started to distance myself from him. I felt a lot of guilt about that decision, and I took my brother's loss very hard.

When I had my intake appointment for the self-help program, I was told I needed more intensive support and was referred to another service provider. I was given an estimate of around four weeks to hear back, but told it could take longer due to COVID-19. After already waiting so long for counselling through our healthcare system, it seemed like paying out of pocket might be the only way to get help in a timely way.

Although I had extended health benefits from my work, they wouldn't go far. Before booking with a counsellor in private practice, I decided to reach out to the perinatal mental health program to see how much longer I might have to wait. It had been about nine months since I requested the referral, and I was shocked to find out I was even not on the waitlist. The clerk I spoke with indicated no referral had ever been received, although I was under the impression from my doctor it had been sent twice.

When I followed up with my doctor's office, I was informed they tried to send the referral but the program was not accepting them at the time. I reached out to the program again, and the clerk advised they did not stop accepting referrals during that time. This left me with many questions: Why did my doctor never inform me the referral was not accepted and I should seek support elsewhere? Was the referral never sent and the office was trying to cover up the oversight? In my discussions with the program, I was told their typical wait time is one to two months, which meant I could have received help already.

At the time of writing, I am still trying to navigate accessing support for postpartum anxiety and grief during this never-ending pandemic. I have an intake appointment scheduled for psychotherapy in a couple of weeks, and I'm hopeful that I'll finally start receiving help. My experience trying to obtain perinatal mental health care during COVID-19 has been both frustrating and disappointing. Mothers are told to speak up when they are struggling but can still fall through the cracks when they do. Concerns might not be taken seriously or help might not be available when it is most needed. I've learned self-advocacy is important but so, too, is advocating for systemic improvements. Now, more than ever, perinatal mental health needs to be taken more seriously by both practitioners and politicians and I'll keep talking about it until they do.

Tanya Nayler is a mom of two and lives in Ottawa. She has worked in law, politics, and public policy. She is also a writer who is passionate about environmental and social justice issues, as well as mental health. You can find Tanya on Twitter @TanyaNayler

CHECKED OUT

Taylor Johnson

PARENTING IS HARD.

Parenting during a global pandemic is really hard.

Parenting a medically complex child during a global pandemic, I would have to say, is the hardest.

How am I supposed to know which category my stress and anxiety fall into? The boxes are blurred and sometimes connect and change shape and size on a daily basis.

Between being a first time mom and dealing with all that entails, I'm also constantly driving to and from the hospital to have my son's nasogastric (NG) feeding tube placed only for him to inevitably pull it out again two days later.

My son also has a bottle aversion, and I'm constantly having to deal with the cancelling and rescheduling of surgery for him. Add to that, the lack of physical support around me due to pandemic restrictions, and yeah, I've hit a wall.

I've completely checked out. I've learned to function at a base level during the hours of screaming. I'm on complete autopilot.

I wake up to a screaming baby. I take said screaming baby downstairs, change his diaper, make a bottle of which he drinks less than an ounce. Then I hook up the NG system and awkwardly hold the feeding tube with one hand while trying to wrangle my screaming and writhing baby with the other.

Shush, I know, but you have to eat. You need to eat. I know it's hard. The looming failure to thrive diagnosis is always hovering over my head. I need to hold him upright for twenty minutes after his feeding and cross my fingers it all stays down.

Next I wash the bottle and NG equipment and have repeated it all, over and over for the last seven months. [Wake up to screaming baby. Take baby downstairs. Change diaper. Make a bottle. He drinks less than an ounce. Hook up NG system. Awkwardly hold feeding tube with one hand while trying to wrangle screaming and writhing baby with the other. *Shush, I know, but you have to eat, you need to eat, I know it's hard.* The looming failure to thrive diagnosis was always hovering over my head. Hold upright for twenty minutes after feed. Cross fingers that it stays down this time. Wash bottle and NG equipment. Repeat over and over and over for seven months.]

I think it's just stress, what I'm feeling.

Everyone goes through this, right? The baby blues? No one tells me that the baby blues really only count for the first month or so. Why is stress hitting me so much harder than any other stress in my life up until this point?

I dealt with multiple diagnoses in my pregnancy and totally rolled with it. A one in 30 chance of developing Trisomy 21? I dealt with it. A high chance of pre-eclampsia and likely low birth weight? I dealt with it. The baby has a heart defect and might have an umbilical cord issue? I dealt with it.

I dealt with it all.

But the level of perfection I expect from myself now that we're home after six weeks in the neonatal intensive care unit was not expected.

At all.

Of course like most new moms, I had this idea of an idyllic first year. It would be wonderful and loving, and I would get to share it with the people around me.

Until the lockdown hit, that is.

I am at least partially thankful that the pandemic came when it did. I have an automatic excuse for not exposing my high-risk baby to those around me. I don't feel guilty for turning down invitations. I am already on leave so I'm not at risk of being laid off.

But it comes with its downfalls, too. I don't get to have the support around me that I would have liked. I don't get to do most of the things I had planned for my perfect year off. I was looking forward to mama and baby yoga and swimming lessons, to visiting my aunt's farm, to travelling up north to see my husband's family. The library! I just wanted to go to the library.

I would hate to go anywhere anyway because it's such a hassle. I would need to remember to pack at least two changes of clothes for him and one for me because he will projectile vomit. I would need to pack the bottle, formula, NG system, pH strips, and sterile water to flush the tube. I would need to know how far away our hospital was from where we were going in case we need to hightail it there. Nope. We're not going anywhere. I would need the phone number of other hospitals as well, because not all nurses have placed infant NGs outside of nursing school (speaking from experience...).

As much as I don't want to, I begin to resent my son for a while.

Feeding becomes more difficult. I find myself getting increasingly angry at him for not eating. I silently cry (sometimes loudly) while trying to make him eat. I am still checked out. I don't realize that I am force feeding him. I don't realize that I am ultimately the cause of him not eating. I am so focused on him eating that I didn't give him a chance to relearn on his own. I am so set on the number and the total ounces required per day based on his weight and the high-density calculations to increase his caloric intake that I lose all my instincts and force him.

My focus is purely on the total amount. Constant mental calculations of how far off he is for the day. He loses trust in me. I don't even know I am doing it until my husband finds me violently sobbing on the bathroom floor holding my son, with the nipple of the bottle shoved so far in his mouth, he is starting to gag and throw up. I don't even know. I am so far gone.

I can't do the most basic thing, feed my child. How could I mess that up? Babies sleep, eat, and poop. That's basically it. Why couldn't I handle one of the three main tasks? I blame myself entirely. I put the entire weight of my son's health on my shoulders and refuse to share the heaviness with anyone, including my husband. I should be able to do it on my own.

I don't realize I may be suffering from postpartum anxiety until I am sitting on the couch at 2 a.m., my tubed son freshly asleep over my shoulder, and open an email from a local university doing a study on anxiety in pregnancy and postpartum. I am four months postpartum, and I decide to do the questionnaire. As I am answering the questions, I am crying in the dark, and it clicks. This is what's wrong. It's not just a little bit of stress. It's not that I'm a failure. It's not me.

It's the whole damn thing. It's postpartum anxiety.

I call the Pacific Postpartum Support Society the next day and sob on the phone to one of the support workers. My public health nurse happens to call the next day, and I sob on the phone with her. I am at my son's pediatrician a week later, and she reminds me that I'm not a failure, that I'm human, and that it's okay to ask for help. Who knew that pediatricians also cared about parents? Maybe I just have a really good one.

My doctor suggested I try medication. We decided on one which is okay to take short or long term in case it wasn't working the way it should. It was a bit of work to get the dosage correct, but I'm so glad I chose the path of medication. I felt like myself again.

The anxiety didn't go away entirely, but it became so much more manageable. I truly had my life back.

I'm thankful for the people who I can lean on while I work my way back to my normal self. I learn to ground myself and to not blame myself when things go wrong. I get myself back into my roll with the punches pregnancy brain brings and just let things happen. I remember that it's okay to be sad and angry and to have moments where you hate your child and your partner and the people around you. Everyone does. It's a matter of getting out of that and moving forward. Life isn't perfect—it's messy and wonderful. I've learned to be okay with what happens, to not blame myself if something goes wrong. It's just another step, and maybe it's a step backwards or sideways or upside down. I just have to step forward when I can.

Taylor Johnson is a mom of one and lives in Burnaby, British Columbia. She works with her husband, running their construction company, and can usually be found taking long walks with a coffee in hand. You can find Taylor on Instagram @taylorrhope

THE PAST, PRESENT, AND FUTURE OF PERINATIAL MENTAL HEALTH

Dr. Jodi Pawluski

OVER THE PAST DECADE THERE has been a growing awareness that becoming a mother isn't always a time of joy and fulfillment. Many birthing people suffer with anxiety, depression, rage, mania and psychosis – particularly in the weeks following birth. Although our understanding and acceptance of perinatal mental illness (i.e. mental illness around the time of birth) is growing there is still a misconception of what and how a mother should be that is often unrealistic and impossible.

Perinatal mental illness, of which there are quite a few, is not a new illness. Pregnant and birthing people have struggled throughout the ages. This news may bring you comfort in knowing that you are not alone. The problem is that perinatal mental illness hasn't received the recognition and understanding that it should have received when our advancements in other areas of mental health have been made. Fortunately, we are starting to recognize what historical texts talked about - that perinatal mental illness is related to physiological changes of childbirth and these changes are often linked to the maternal brain.

Throughout the ages mental illness around the time of childbirth has been recorded, albeit periodically, with particular emphasis on those severe cases marked by delirium and mania. The first written record of postpartum mental illness is attributed to Hippocrates in 400 B.C. where he provides brief descriptions of 8-9 cases of postpartum delirium or mania in his book titled Epidemics. One such description reads as follows: "In Cyzicus a woman gave birth with a difficult labour to twin daughters....First day. Acute fever with shivering; painful heaviness of the head and neck. Sleepless from the first...Sixth day. Much wandering at night; no sleep. About the eleventh day she went out of her mind and then was rational again...Fourteenth day. Many convulsions; extremities cold; no further recovery of reason; urine suppressed. Sixteenth day. Speechless. Seventeenth day. Death.

From these early records of postpartum mental illness by Hippocrates the new mothers that suffered from delirium or mania appeared to do so as a consequence of a severe infection and fever. This is something we now call puerperal fever and because it is due to an infection it is not considered a typical postpartum mental illness of modern day. Nonetheless, there are three things that I find striking about Hippocrates' early descriptions of postpartum delirium. First, he acknowledged a link between birth and mental illness - Thank you! Today we know that the immediate postpartum period is a time in a woman's life when she is at the greatest risk of being hospitalized for a mental illness. Second, his writings show a link between what we know now as immune function, as evidenced by fever in the women he described, and delirium. Today we are starting to understand how that immune system may be linked to postpartum mental illness in the absence of infection and fever. Third, he proposed that the brain is a key source of mental illness postpartum. Hippocrates predicted that lochial discharge—the fluid that comes from the uterus after birth - if suppressed, could flow to the head and result in agitation, delirium and attacks of mania. With our advances in neuroscience we know this exact scenario doesn't exist, but brain changes are definitely involved in all perinatal mental illness—during the postpartum and during pregnancy.

But I'm getting ahead of myself, let's continue on the history of perinatal mental illness. After Hippocrates the next known reference to a perinatal mental illness was by Trotula of Salerno, an 11th century professor of medicine or a 13th century midwife, who wrote: "If the womb is too moist, the brain is filled with water, and the moisture running over the eyes, compels them to involuntarily shed tears."

This is a rather beautiful description of postpartum depression. The brain is full of water that it must release and this is done through crying. Like Hippocrates, Trotula attributed postpartum mental illness to fluid buildup in the brain—noting, again, the importance of the connection between bodily fluids and the brain in mental illness after birth.

In the Middle Ages, the idea of perinatal mental illness began to change and it appears that mental illnesses not attributed to fever or infection in the new mother were talked about. These perinatal mental illnesses were referred to as disturbances of the 'maternal instinct' in new mothers and ranged from melancholia or feelings of deep sadness, hatred of the newborn and, in extreme cases, infant abuse and infanticide. In 1547, a Portuguese physician practicing in Rome, Joao Rodrigues de Casello Branco, gives a brief description of postpartum melancholia as follows: "The beautiful wife of Carcinator (a merchant) who always enjoyed the best of health, was attacked after childbirth by melancholy, and remained insane for a month, but recovered with treatment." Note that recovery was not always that quick or easy. There are records of postpartum melancholy leading to suicide and "depressive filicide."

Society in the Middle Ages was also not understanding of these disturbances of 'maternal instinct' and often mothers who exhibited such 'disturbances' were said to be witches or had dabbled in witchcraft. This is not a surprise as many stigmatized individuals of the day, and often women, were considered witches and likely burned at the stake or subject to whatever punishment was the current fashion. When I was 12 I went to Edinburgh, Scotland and during a tour I remember being told that during the Middle Ages if a woman was considered a witch she was thrown into the river. If she survived there was no doubt that she was a witch and she would then be burned at the stake. If she drowned in the river she was not a witch. This was obviously a lose-lose situation. Thankfully we don't physically burn mothers at the stake today if they lack 'maternal instinct' but too often we do stigmatize mothers as 'bad mothers' - so perhaps we haven't changed that much?

Disturbances of 'maternal instinct' up until the 1800s often referred to postpartum melancholia and delirium. However, anxiety and obsessions in new mothers were also written about as early as the 1600s, but they did not get the attention they deserved at the time.

It wasn't until the mid-1800s that we began to see an acknowledgement of the impact of pregnancy, birth, and postpartum on mental health in birthing people outside of fever-induced delirium. Interestingly these 'maternal conditions' were not always considered mental maladies, especially when it came to psychosis and infanticide, but were considered part of forensic medicine—"an area of medicine dealing with the application of medical knowledge to establish facts in civil or criminal legal cases, such as an investigation into the cause and time of a suspicious death". Take for example one of the first non-fever-related postpartum delirium cases written about by Jean-Etienne Esquirol, a Parisian physician, in 1845. Note he does not see this case fitting for his book on mental maladies:

"Neither will I speak of the delirium of those who, in their phrens, destroy the children to whom they have just given birth. False shame, perplexity, fear, misery and crime, do not always lead to infanticide. Delirium however, by disturbing the reason of the recently confined, sometimes also, directs their sacrilegious hands. A maiden becomes pregnant, does not conceal the fact...and announces the expected event to all. She is confined during the night. On the following day, she is found in her bed and the child in the privy [dead from stabbing]... Has not this young woman suffered from an attack of delirium? Finally, this and other facts of similar import, belong to legal medicine, and ought not to occupy me here ."

It wasn't until 1858 when Louis Marcé, a French physician, who studied under Esquirol, wrote an entire book on psychiatric disorders of women during and following pregnancy. The book titled Traité de la folie des femmes enceintes was the first of its kind and recorded illnesses during the entire transition to motherhood; throughout pregnancy and postpartum.

When writing about mental illnesses in pregnancy, Marcé notes that the most common mental illness during this time is depression (melancholia) and that mania and manic-depressive symptoms can also be evident. He also noted that the symptoms of these mental illnesses decreased as pregnancy progressed, something we're not clear about today. What I find interesting is that Marcé didn't view pregnancy as a time of joy and fulfillment, especially for those women with pre-existing mental illness. At the time, physicians were prescribing pregnancy as a treatment for women who suffered from mental maladies and Marcé was very much against this practice, rightfully so. He knew that pregnancy did not always make a woman happy. [And, by the way, when did we start to think that pregnancy and motherhood were analogous to happiness?]

Marcé recorded that postpartum mental illnesses were the most frequent and severe of all perinatal "insanities." He wrote about mania, melancholia, delusional states, and other psychotic illnesses and noted that they sometimes showed unusual features postpartum compared to other times in life. He acknowledged the complexity of these postpartum disorders and the fact that they may not occur during the immediate postpartum but could become evident months later. Although he doesn't remark much on perinatal anxiety specifically, he does note that: "Where subjects [women] are predisposed to mental illness through either hereditary antecedents, previous illnesses, or through an excessive nervous susceptibility, pregnancy, delivery and lactation can have disastrous repercussions."

Marcé's comprehensive text on perinatal mental illness didn't get the recognition that it deserved when published in 1858 but his legacy has lived on. Perhaps his name is most recognized in The International Marcé Society for Perinatal Mental Health, an "interdisciplinary organization dedicated to supporting research and assistance surrounding prenatal and postpartum mental health for mothers, fathers and their babies". I'd like to think that Marcé would be astonished by what he has inspired.

In the late 1800s, Emil Kraepelin, a German physician, wrote more about the relationship between childbirth-related psychiatric disorders and, particularly, manic-depressive illness. He writes that amentia "... an acute state of dreamlike confusion, illusionary or hallucinatory distortion of reality and motor agitation" often occurs after childbirth. We would likely refer to amentia as postpartum psychosis today but Kraepelin also described amentia as being accompanied by depressed mood, thus pointing to a bipolar disorder. Kraepelin stressed that child birth is a potent trigger for mood episodes in women but also noted that pregnancy could have a protective effect against depression in some patients with manic-depressive illness. Interestingly there is research today supporting these first ideas that pregnancy can have positive effects on the course of bipolar disorder in some women.

As with Marcé, Kraepelin's work on the role of pregnancy and the postpartum period on perinatal manic-depressive illness was overlooked but many but his descriptions and ideas hold true today. For example, key points from Kraepelin's work showed that birth, lack of sleep and a history of a mental illness were contributing factors to the onset of postpartum manic-depressive illness. These are all factors we know from current research can increase the risk of developing symptoms of bipolar disorder postpartum.

In the mid to late 1900s a champion of perinatal mental health was Channi Kumar, a psychiatrist in London, England. He is a key figure in the development of perinatal psychiatry as a specialty and was internationally recognized for his research into the causes, consequences and treatment of postpartum mental illness. One of Kumar's greatest achievements was in raising awareness—in public, medical and academic arenas—about postpartum mental illness and its impact on mothers, their babies and family. He was also a founding member of the International Marcé Society, mentioned earlier.

As you can see, throughout history a number of men have championed our current understanding of perinatal mental illness but more recently warriors and sheros have come to the forefront from a range of professional backgrounds and with lived experience. Some women leading the way to improving awareness and treatments of perinatal mental illnesses that come to my mind today are Dr. Katherine Wisner, Karen Kleiman (Founder of The Postpartum Stress Center), Dr. Samantha Meltzer-Brody, Alanis Morrisette, and Chrissy Teigen. Luckily, there are too many sheros to name here as the field of perinatal mental health has continued to expand exponentially over the years.

But where do we go from here? The first records of postpartum mental illness linked causes of these disorders to bodily fluids and the effect of these fluids on the brain. These ideas were ahead of their time and current research is starting to show that, indeed, changes in the maternal brain during pregnancy and the postpartum period are related to perinatal mental illnesses. These perinatal mental illnesses are very much biological events that are linked to neuroscience, experience and physiology. They are treatable illnesses. As our research and understanding improves we can add to our growing list of interventions and preventative measures to improve the lives of so many mothers who suffer in silence. But advances in improving perinatal mental health can only be made when governments, research institutions, health care providers, scientists and the general public see the mental health of birthing people as a priority.

For those pregnancy and postpartum persons who are struggling, there is hope, things are changing and as the universal message from

Postpartum Support International states - You are not alone, you are not to blame, and with help you will be well.

Dr. Jodi Pawluski is a neuroscientist studying how stress and stress-related disorders, such as anxiety and depression, affect the maternal brain during pregnancy and the postpartum. Her research supports the idea that if antidepressant medications are effective in treating maternal mood and anxiety symptoms during pregnancy a mom should continue to use them. Jodi also hosts the podcast, Mommy Brain Revisited and works as a therapist for women. She is originally from the Okanagan Valley but is based in France where she lives with her husband, two kids, three sheep, two plus cats and a few chickens. You can get in touch with Jodi at www.jodipawluski.com.

ACKNOWLEDGMENTS

WE'D FIRST AND FOREMOST LIKE to thank each and every person that submitted a story for this anthology. Please know that each and every word, phrase, and story was pored over again and again, and we are so thankful for the time and effort each one of you spent in telling your story. We would have loved to include them all. Perhaps we need to think about extending this anthology into a series and publish more in volume two! Please know that we truly appreciate your willingness to share your story and whether we proceed with more anthologies or not, we will be in touch to share your story in some way, shape and form.

We'd like to thank our publisher, Heather Down, of Wintertickle Press and her team for supporting our vision and mission and for enthusiastically walking with us down this path.

Thank you to our experts who agreed whole-heartedly to contribute chapters for our anthology on tight deadlines, knowing that you already have so much work and other commitments on your plate. We are so grateful for your belief in us and our project.

And one last huge thank you to our National Committee and Social Media Ambassadors of the Canadian Perinatal Mental Health Collaborative for their insight and advice on how to make the anthology as inclusive and helpful as possible.

RESOURCES

PLEASE NOTE THAT THESE RESOURCES were available at time of publication. However, Wintertickle Press cannot take responsibility if these resources become unavailable. If you are in crisis, please seek out medical attention immediately.

INTERNATIONAL:

Postpartum Support International

www.postpartum.net

Text: 503-894-9453

World Maternal Mental Health Day

www.wmmhd.postpartum.net

CANADA:

Canadian Perinatal Mental Health Collaborative

www.cpmhc.ca

Pacific Post Partum Support Society

www.postpartum.org

Text: 604-255-7999

Women's College Hospital, Reproductive Life Stages Program

www.womenscollegehospital.ca

Phone: 416-323-7715

Mount Sinai Hospital, Perinatal Mental Health Program

www.mountsinai.on.ca

Phone: 416-586-4800, ext. 8325

U.S.

Postpartum Stress Center
www.postpartumstress.com
Phone: 610-525-7527

2020 Mom
www.2020mom.org
Phone: 310-955-1081

Maternal Mental Health Leadership Alliance
www.mmhla.org
Phone: 571-643-2738

UNITED KINGDOM

Action on Postpartum Psychosis
www.app-network.org

Maternal Mental Health Alliance
www.maternalmentalhealthalliance.org

AUSTRALIA

PANDA, Perinatal Anxiety & Depression Australia
www.panda.org.au
National Helpline: 1300 726 306

CONNECT

Do you have a story to share? If you would like your story to be considered for future editions of *You are Not Alone*, please email your story idea to canpmhc@gmail.com and be sure to follow us on social media!

Facebook: Canadian Perinatal Mental Health Collaborative

Twitter: @canpmhc

Instagram: @cpmhc

REFERENCES

INCLUSIVITY

1. Canadian Association of Midwives. (2015). A Statement on Gender Inclusivity & Human Rights. CAM. Retrieved from https://canadianmidwives.org/wp-content/uploads/2016/06/CAM-GenderInclusivity-HumanRights-Sept2015.pdf

2. Bonifacio, J. (2017). Creating inclusive spaces for the LGBTTQ+ community: Learning from the experts. Society of Obstetricians and Gynaecologists of Canada (SOGC) News. Retrieved from https://d3n8a8pro7vhmx.cloudfront.net/acc/pages/190/attachments/original/1508448414/SOGC_11381_Newsletter_September_FINAL.pdf?1508448414

3. Veltman, A., & Chaimowitz, G. (2014). Position Paper: Mental Health Care for People Who Identify as Lesbian, Gay, Bisexual, Transgender, and (or) Queer. The Canadian Journal of Psychiatry, 59(11). Retrieved from https://www.cpa-apc.org/wp-content/uploads/LGBTQ-2014-55-web-FIN-EN.pdf

4. MacDonald, T., et al. (2016). Transmasculine individuals' experiences with lactation, chestfeeding, and gender identity: a qualitative study. BMC Pregnancy Childbirth, 16(106).

5. Nelson, M., et al. (2020). Beyond the binary: What does gender-inclusive women's health research look like? Women's Health Research Institute at BC Women's. Retrieved from https://whri.org/beyond-the-binary-what-does-gender-inclusive-womens-health-research-look-like/

6. Midwives Alliance North America. (2015). Use of Inclusive Language. MANA. Retrieved from https://mana.org/healthcare-policy/use-of-inclusive-language

7. Meyer I.H. (2003). Prejudice, social stress, and mental health in lesbian, gay, and bisexual populations: conceptual issues and research evidence. Psychological Bulletin, 129(5), 674-697.

8. Valdiserri, R.O., et al. (2019). Unraveling Health Disparities Among Sexual and Gender Minorities: A Commentary on the Persistent Impact of Stigma. Journal of Homosexuality, 66(5), 571-589.

9. Khan, M., et al. (2017). Multifactorial discrimination as a fundamental cause of mental health inequities. International Journal for Equity in Health, 16(1).

10. Lee, J.H., et al. (2016). Discrimination, Mental Health, and Substance Use Disorders Among Sexual Minority Populations. LGBT Health, 3(4), 258-265.

11. Steele, L.S., et al. (2009). Women's Sexual Orientation and Health: Results from a Canadian Population-Based Survey. Women & Health, 49(5), 353-367.

12. Ross, L.E., et al. (2018). Prevalence of Depression and Anxiety Among Bisexual People Compared to Gay, Lesbian, and Heterosexual Individuals: A Systematic Review and Meta-Analysis. The Journal of Sex Research, 55(4-5), 435-456.

13. Rotondi, N.K., et al. (2012). Prevalence of and Risk and Protective Factors for Depression in Female-to-Male Transgender Ontarians: Trans PULSE Project. Canadian Journal of Community Mental Health, 30(2), 135-155.

14. MacLeod, M.A., et al. (2015). Biphobia and Anxiety among Bisexuals in Ontario, Canada. Journal of Gay & Lesbian Mental Health, 19(3), 217-243.

15. Salway, T., et al. (2019). A Systematic Review and Meta-Analysis of Disparities in the Prevalence of Suicide Ideation and Attempt among Bisexual Populations. Archives of Sexual Behavior, 48(1), 89-111.

16. Abramovich, A., et al. (2020). Assessment of Health Conditions and Health Service Use among Transgender Patients in Canada. JAMA Network Open, 3(8).

17. Borgogna, N.C., et al. (2019). Anxiety and depression across gender and sexual minorities: Implications for transgender, gender nonconforming, pansexual, demisexual, asexual, queer, and questioning individuals. Psychology of Sexual Orientation and Gender Diversity, 6(1), 54-63.

18. Winter, S., et al. (2016). Transgender people: health at the margins of society. The Lancet, 388(10042), 390-400.

19. Greenfield, M. & Darwin, Z. (2020) Trans and non-binary pregnancy, traumatic birth, and perinatal mental health: a scoping review. International Journal of Transgender Health.

20. Ross, L.E., et al. (2018). Bisexuality: The Invisible Sexual Orientation in Sexual and Reproductive Health Care. Journal of Obstetrics and Gynaecology Canada, 40(8), 1057-1060.

21. Flanders, C.E., et al. (2016). Postpartum depression among visible and invisible sexual minority women: a pilot study. Archives of Women's Mental Health, 19, 299-305.

22. Ross, L., et al. (2007). Perinatal depressive symptomatology among lesbian and bisexual women. Archives of Women's Mental Health, 10, 53-59.

23. Ross, L.E., et al. (2012). "I Don't Want to Turn Totally Invisible": Mental Health, Stressors, and Supports among Bisexual Women during the Perinatal Period. Journal of GLBT Family Studies, 8(2), 137-154.

24. Besse, M., et al. (2020). Focus: Sex & Reproduction: Experiences with Achieving Pregnancy and Giving Birth among Transgender Men: A Narrative Literature Review. The Yale Journal of Biology and Medicine, 93(4), 517-528.

25. Snow, A., et al. (2019). Barriers to Mental Health Care for Transgender and Gender-Nonconforming Adults: A Systematic Literature Review. Health & Social Work, 44(3), 149-155.

26. Jaffee, K.D., et al. (2016). Discrimination and Delayed Health Care among Transgender Women and Men: Implications for Improving Medical Education and Health Care Delivery. Medical Care, 54(11), 1010-1016.

27. Kcomt, L., et al. (2020). Healthcare avoidance due to anticipated discrimination among transgender people: A call to create trans-affirmative environments. SSM-Population Health, 11.

28. van Dam, M.A.A., et al. (2001). Lesbian Disclosure to Health Care Providers and Delay of Care. Journal of the Gay and Lesbian Medical Association, 5, 11-19.

29. Bauer, G.R., et al. (2014). Reported emergency department avoidance, use, and experiences of transgender persons in Ontario, Canada: Results from a respondent-driven sampling survey. Annals of Emergency Medicine, 63(6), 713-720.

30. Seelman, K.L., et al. (2017). Transgender Noninclusive Healthcare and Delaying Care Because of Fear: Connections to General Health and Mental Health among Transgender Adults. Transgender Health, 2(1), 17-28.

31. Abelsohn K.A., et al. (2013). Celebrating the "Other" Parent: Mental Health and Wellness of Expecting Lesbian, Bisexual, and Queer Non-Birth Parents. Journal of Gay & Lesbian Mental Health, 17(4), 387-405.

32. Cameron, E.E., et al. (2016). Prevalence of paternal depression in pregnancy and the postpartum: An updated meta-analysis. Journal of Affective Disorders, 206, 189-203.

33. Da Costa, D., et al. (2017). Dads Get Sad Too: Depressive Symptoms and Associated Factors in Expectant First-Time Fathers. American Journal of Men's Health, 11(5), 1376-1384.

34. Singh G.K. (2021). Trends and Social Inequalities in Maternal Mortality in the United States, 1969-2018. International Journal of MCH and AIDS, 10(1), 29-42.

35. Vedam, S., et al. (2019). The Giving Voice to Mothers study: Inequity and mistreatment during pregnancy and childbirth in the United States. Reproductive Health, 16(77).

36. Mitra, M., et al. (2015). Prevalence and risk factors for postpartum depression symptoms among women with disabilities. Maternal and Child Health Journal, 19(2), 362-372.

37. Black, K.A., et al. (2019). Postpartum Mental Health Disorders in Indigenous Women: A Systematic Review and Meta-Analysis. Journal of Obstetrics and Gynaecology Canada, 41(10), 1470-1478.

38. Miller, F. (2020). Why Inclusive Language Matters in Medicine. Op-Med. Retrieved from https://opmed.doximity.com/articles/why-inclusive-language-matters-in-medicine

MOTHERHOOD< ANXIETY, AND SCARY THOUGHTS

Abramowitz, J., Khandker, M., Nelson, C., Deacon, B., & Rygwall, R. (2006). The role of cognitive factors in the pathogenesis of obsessive-compulsive symptoms: a prospective study. Behav Res Ther. 2006 Sep;44(9):1361-74. doi: 10.1016/j.brat.2005.09.011.

Choi, K., Chen, C., & Stein, M., et al. (2019). Assessment of bidirectional relationships between physical activity and depression among adults. A 2-sample Mendelian randomization study. JAMA Psychiatry. 1;76(4):399-408.

Fairbrother, N., & Woody, S. (2008). New mothers' thoughts of harm related to the newborn. Archives of Women's Mental Health, 11(3), 221-229. doi:10.1007/s00737-008-0016-7.

Kabat-Zinn J. (2003). Mindfulness-based interventions in context: Past, present and future. Clinical Psychology: Science and Practice, 10(2), 144–156. https://doi.org/10.1093/clipsy.bpg016

Kleiman, K. (2019). Good Moms Have Scary Thoughts: A Healing Guide to the Secret Fears of New Mothers. (Familius: Sanger, CA).

Kleiman, K., Wenzel, A., Waller, H., & Adler-Mandel, A. (2020). Dropping the Baby and Other Scary Thoughts: Breaking the Cycle of Unwanted Thoughts in Parenthood (Second Edition.) Routledge: New York.

Zane, M. & Milt, H. (1984) Your Phobia: Understanding Your Fears Through Contextual Therapy. American Psychiatric Press.

HOW COMMON IS POST PARTUM ANGER?

Arendell, T. (2000). Conceiving and investigating motherhood: The decade's scholarship. Journal of Marriage and Family, 62(4), 1192-1207. doi:10.1111/j.1741-3737.2000.01192.x

Asgeirsdottir, B. B., & Sigfusdottir, I. D. (2015). Gender differences in co-occurrence of depressive and anger symptoms among adolescents in five Nordic countries. Scandinavian journal of public health, 43(2), 183-189.

Averill, J. R. (1982). Anger and aggression: An essay on emotion. New York, NY: Springer New York. doi:10.1007/978-1-4612-5743-1

Beck, C. T. (2002). Postpartum depression: A metasynthesis. Qualitative Health Research, 12(4), 453-472. doi:10.1177/104973202129120016

Beck, C. T. (2015). Middle range theory of traumatic childbirth: The ever-widening ripple effect. Global Qualitative Nursing Research, 2, 2333393615575313-2333393615575313. doi:10.1177/2333393615575313

Bruno, A., Laganà, A. S., Leonardi, V., Greco, D., Merlino, M., Vitale, S. G., ... & Muscatello, M. R. A. (2017). Inside–out: the role of anger experience and expression in the development of postpartum mood disorders. The Journal of Maternal-Fetal & Neonatal Medicine, 1-6.

CassiellomRobbins, C., & Barlow, D. H. (2016). Anger: The unrecognized emotion in emotional disorders. Clinical Psychology: Science and Practice, 23(1), 66-85. doi:10.1111/cpsp.12139

Chemaly, S. L. (2018). Rage becomes her: The power of women's anger (First Atria Books hardcover ed.). New York: Atria Books.

DiGiuseppe, R., & Tafrate, R. C. (2007;2006;). Understanding anger disorders. New York: Oxford University Press. doi:10.1093/med:psych/9780195170795.001.0001

Ellsworth, P. C., & Tong, E. M. (2006). What does it mean to be angry at yourself? Categories, appraisals, and the problem of language. Emotion, 6(4), 572.

Flake, E. (2018). "Parent" as a verb: Mommy rage. New Yorker Magazine. Retrieved from: https://www.newyorker.com/culture/culture-desk/parent-as-a-verb-mommy-rage

Field, T., Diego, M., Hernandez-Reif, M., Schanberg, S., Kuhn, C., Yando, R., & Bendell, D. (2003). Pregnancy anxiety and comorbid depression and anger: Effects on the fetus and neonate. Depression and Anxiety, 17(3), 140-151. doi:10.1002/da.10071

Field, T., Hernandez-Reif, M., Vera, Y., Gil, K., Diego, M., Bendell, D., & Yando, R. (2005). Anxiety and anger effects on depressed mother–infant spontaneous and imitative interactions. Infant Behavior and Development, 28(1), 1-9.

Germer, C. K., & Neff, K. D. (2013). Self-compassion in clinical practice. Journal of Clinical Psychology, 69(8), 856-867. doi:10.1002/jclp.22021

Kettunen, P. Koistinen, E., & Hintikka, J. (2014). Is postpartum depression a homogenous disorder: Time of onset, severity, symptoms and hopelessness in relation to the course of depression. BMC Pregnancy and Childbirth, 14(1), 402. doi:10.1186/PREACCEPT-1201881224127235

Klein, M. H. Hyde, J. S., Essex, M. J., & Clark, R. (1998). Maternity leave, role quality, work involvement, and mental health one year after delivery. Psychology of Women Quarterly, 22(2), 239-266.

Krizan, Z., & Hisler, G. (2019). Sleepy anger: Restricted sleep amplifies angry feelings. Journal of Experimental Psychology, 148(7), 1239.

Martin, R. C., & Dahlen, E. R. (2005). Cognitive emotion regulation in the prediction of depression, anxiety, stress, and anger. Personality and Individual Differences, 39(7), 1249-1260. doi:10.1016/j.paid.2005.06.004

Monteiro, F., Fonseca, A., Pereira, M., Alves, S., & Canavarro, M. C. (2019). What protects at-risk postpartum women from developing depressive and anxiety symptoms? The role of acceptance-focused processes and self-compassion. Journal of Affective Disorders, 246, 522-529.

Ou, C. H., & Hall, W. A. (2018). Anger in the context of postnatal depression: An integrative review. Birth. Advanced Online Publication. doi.org/10.1111/birt.12356

Potegal, M., Stemmler, G., Spielberger, C. D. (2010). International handbook of anger: Constituent and concomitant biological, psychological, and social processes (1st ed.). New York: Springer.

Simon, R. W., & Lively, K. (2010). Sex, anger and depression. Social Forces, 88(4), 1543-1568.

Tavris, C. (1989). Anger: The misunderstood emotion (Rev. ed.). New York: Simon & Schuster.

Vliegen, N., Casalin, S., Luyten, P., Docx, R., Lenaerts, M., Tang, E., & Kempke, S. (2013). Hospitalization-based treatment for postpartum depressed mothers and their babies: rationale, principles, and preliminary follow-up data. Psychiatry: Interpersonal & Biological Processes, 76(2), 150-168.

POSTPARTUM PSYCHOSIS

1 National Institute for Health and Care Excellence (2018). Antenatal and postnatal mental health: Clinical management and service guidance. [National Clinical Guideline Number 192).https://www.nice.org.uk/guidance/cg192/evidence/full-guideline-pdf-4840896925

2 Heron, J., McGuinness, M., Blackmore, E. R., Craddock, N., & Jones, I. (2008). Early postpartum symptoms in puerperal psychosis. BJOG: An International Journal of Obstetrics & Gynaecology, 115(3), 348-353.

3 Valdimarsdóttir, U., Hultman, C. M., Harlow, B., Cnattingius, S., & Sparén, P. (2009). Psychotic illness in first-time mothers with no previous psychiatric hospitalizations: a population-based study. PLoS Med, 6(2), e1000013.

4 VanderKruik, R., Barreix, M., Chou, D., Allen, T., Say, L., Cohen, L.S., & Maternal Morbidity Working Group. (2017). The global prevalence of postpartum psychosis: A systematic review. BMC Psychiatry, 17, 272.

5 Arifin, S. R. M., Cheyne, H., & Maxwell, M (2018). Review of the prevalence of postnatal depression across cultures. AIMS Public Health, 5(3): 260-295.

6 Munk-Olsen, T., Laursen, T. M., Pedersen, C. B., Mors, O., & Mortensen, P. B. (2006). New parents and mental disorders: A population-based register study. JAMA, 296(21), 2582-2589.

7 Berrisford, G., Lambert, A., & Heron, J. (2015). Understanding postpartum psychosis. Community Practitioner, 88(5), 22-24.

8 Bergink. V., Rasgon, N., & Wisner, K. L. (2016). Postpartum psychosis: madness, mania, and melancholia in motherhood. American Journal of Psychiatry, 173(12), 1179-1188.

9 Ramsauer, B., & Achtergarde, S. (2018). Mothers with acute and chronic postpartum psychoses and impact on the mother-infant interaction. Schizophrenia Research, 197, 45-58.

10 National Health Service. (2020). Postpartum psychosis. Retrieved on 8/12/2020 from https://www.nhs.uk/conditions/post-partum-psychosis/

11 Kamperman, A. M., Veldman Hoek, M. J., Wesseloo, R., Robertson Blackmore, E., & Bergink, V. (2017). Phenotypical characteristics of postpartum psychosis: A clinical cohort study. Bipolar Disorders, 19(6), 450-457.

12 Kapfhammer, H. P., & Lange, P. (2012). Suizidale und infantizide Risiken im Wochenbett–klinische Erfahrungen bei Frauen mit Puerperalpsychose eines frühen Beginns. Neuropsychiatrie, 26(3), 129-138.

13 Jones, I. & Smith, S. (2009). Puerperal psychosis: identifying and caring for women at risk. Advances in Psychiatric Treatment, 15(6), 411-418.

14 Jones, I. Chandra, P. S., Dazzan, P., & Howard, L. M. (2014). Bipolar disorder, affective psychosis, and schizophrenia in pregnancy and the post-partum period. The Lancet, 384(9956), 1789-1799.

15 Upadhyaya, S. K., Sharma, A., & Raval, C. M. (2014). Postpartum psychosis: Risk factors identification. North American Journal of Medical Sciences, 6(6), 274-277.

16 Nager, A., Sundquist, K., Ramírez-León, V., & Johansson, L. M. (2008). Obstetric complications and postpartum psychosis: a follow-up study of 1.1 million first-time mothers between 1975 and 2003 in Sweden. Acta Psychiatrica Scandinavica, 117(1), 12-19.

17 Aas, M., Vecchio, C., Pauls, A., Mehta, M., Williams, S., Hazelgrove, K., ...& Dazzan, P. (2020). Biological stress response in women at risk of postpartum psychosis: The role of life events and inflammation. Psychoneuroendocrinology, 113, 1-7.

18 Robertson, E., Jones, I., Haque, S., Holder, R., & Craddock, N. (2005). Risk of puerperal and non-puerperal recurrence of illness following bipolar affective puerperal (post-partum) psychosis. The British Journal of Psychiatry, 186(3), 258-259.

19 Davies, W. (2017). Understanding the pathophysiology of postpartum psychosis: Challenges and new approaches. World Journal of Psychiatry, 7(2), 77-88.

20 Jones, I. & Craddock, N. (2007). Searching for the Puerperal Trigger: Molecular Genetic Studies of Bipolar Affective Puerperal Psychosis. Psychopharmacology Bulletin, 40, 2, 115-128.

21 Wittkowski, A., & Santos, N. (2017). Psychological and psychosocial interventions promoting mother-infant interaction on mother and baby units in the United Kingdom. JSM Anxiety Depression, 2(1).

22 Bugerhout, K.M., Kamperman, A.M., Roza, S.J., Lambregtse-Van den Berg, M.P., Koorengevel, K.M., Hoodendijk, W.J.G., ... & Bergink, V. (2016). Functional Recovery After Postpartum Psychosis: A Prospective Longitudinal Study. The Journal of Clinical Psychiatry, 78(1), 122-128.

23 Forde, R., Peters, S., & Wittkowski, A. (2020). Recovery for postpartum psychosis: A systematic review and metasynthesis of women's and families' experiences. Archives of Women's Mental Health, 23, 597-612.

24 Forde, R., Peters, S., Wittkowski, A. (2019). Psychological interventions for managing postpartum psychosis: A qualitative analysis of women's and family members' experiences and preferences. BMC Psychiatry, 19(411), 1-17.

25 Plunkett, C., Peters, S., Wieck, A., & Wittkowski. A. (2017). A qualitative investigation in the role of the baby in recovery from postpartum psychosis. Clinical Psychology & Psychotherapy, 24(5), 1099-1108.

26 Plunkett, C., Peters, S., & Wittkowski, A. (2016). Mothers' experiences of recovery from postnatal mental illness: A systematic review of the qualitative literature and metasynthesis. JSM Anxiety and Depression, 1(4).

27 McGrath, L., Peters, S., Wieck, A., & Wittkowski, A. (2013). The process of recovery in women who experienced psychosis following childbirth. BMC Psychiatry, 13, 341.

28 Bergink, V., Burgerhout, K. M., Koorengevel, K.M., Kamperman, A.M., Hoogendijk, W.J., Lambregtse-van den Berg, M.P. & Kushner, S.A. (2015). Treatment of Psychosis and Mania in the Postpartum Period. Treatment in Psychiatry, 172(2), 115-123.

29 Doucet, S. Jones, I., Letourneau, N., Dennis, C. L., & Blackmore, E. R. (2011). Interventions for the prevention and treatment of postpartum psychosis: a systematic review. Archives of Women's Mental Health, 14(2), 89-98.

30 Gillham, R., & Wittkowski, A. (2015). Outcomes for women admitted to a mother and baby unit: A systematic review. International Journal of Women's Health, 7, 459-476.

31 Hill, R., Law, D., Yelland, C., & Sved Williams, A. (2019). Treatment of postpartum psychosis in a mother-baby unit: do both mother and baby benefit? Australasian Psychiatry, 27(2), 121-124.

32 Teodorescu, A., Dima, L., Popa, M.A., Moga, M.A., Bîgiu, N.F., & Ifteni, P. (2020). Antipsychotics in Postpartum Psychosis. American Journal of Therapeutics, 0(0), 1-8.

HOW COMMON IS POSTPARTUM ANGER?

Arendell, T. (2000). Conceiving and investigating motherhood: The decade's scholarship. Journal of Marriage and Family, 62(4), 1192-1207. doi:10.1111/j.1741-3737.2000.01192.x

Asgeirsdottir, B. B., & Sigfusdottir, I. D. (2015). Gender differences in co-occurrence of depressive and anger symptoms among adolescents in five Nordic countries. Scandinavian journal of public health, 43(2), 183-189.

Averill, J. R. (1982). Anger and aggression: An essay on emotion. New York, NY: Springer New York. doi:10.1007/978-1-4612-5743-1

Beck, C. T. (2002). Postpartum depression: A metasynthesis. Qualitative Health Research, 12(4), 453-472. doi:10.1177/104973202129120016

Beck, C. T. (2015). Middle range theory of traumatic childbirth: The ever-widening ripple effect. Global Qualitative Nursing Research, 2, 2333393615575313-2333393615575313. doi:10.1177/2333393615575313

Bruno, A., Laganà, A. S., Leonardi, V., Greco, D., Merlino, M., Vitale, S. G., ... & Muscatello, M. R. A. (2017). Inside–out: the role of anger experience and expression in the development of postpartum mood disorders. The Journal of Maternal-Fetal & Neonatal Medicine, 1-6.

Cassiellom Robbins, C., & Barlow, D. H. (2016). Anger: The unrecognized emotion in emotional disorders. Clinical Psychology: Science and Practice, 23(1), 66-85. doi:10.1111/cpsp.12139

Chemaly, S. L. (2018). Rage becomes her: The power of women's anger (First Atria Books hardcover ed.). New York: Atria Books.

DiGiuseppe, R., & Tafrate, R. C. (2007;2006;). Understanding anger disorders. New York: Oxford University Press. doi:10.1093/med:psych/9780195170795.001.0001

Ellsworth, P. C., & Tong, E. M. (2006). What does it mean to be angry at yourself? Categories, appraisals, and the problem of language. Emotion, 6(4), 572.

Flake, E. (2018). "Parent" as a verb: Mommy rage. New Yorker Magazine. Retrieved from: https://www.newyorker.com/culture/culture-desk/parent-as-a-verb-mommy-rage

Field, T., Diego, M., Hernandez Reif, M., Schanberg, S., Kuhn, C., Yando, R., & Bendell, D. (2003). Pregnancy anxiety and comorbid depression and anger: Effects on the fetus and neonate. Depression and Anxiety, 17(3), 140-151. doi:10.1002/da.10071

Field, T., Hernandez-Reif, M., Vera, Y., Gil, K., Diego, M., Bendell, D., & Yando, R. (2005). Anxiety and anger effects on depressed mother–infant spontaneous and imitative interactions. Infant Behavior and Development, 28(1), 1-9.

Germer, C. K., & Neff, K. D. (2013). Self-compassion in clinical practice. Journal of Clinical Psychology, 69(8), 856-867. doi:10.1002/jclp.22021

Kettunen, P., Koistinen, E., & Hintikka, J. (2014). Is postpartum depression a homogenous disorder: Time of onset, severity, symptoms and hopelessness in relation to the course of depression. BMC Pregnancy and Childbirth, 14(1), 402. doi:10.1186/PREACCEPT-1301881224127235

Klein, M. H., Hyde, J. S., Essex, M. J., & Clark, R. (1998). Maternity leave, role quality, work involvement, and mental health one year after delivery. Psychology of Women Quarterly, 22(2), 239-266.

Krizan, Z., & Hisler, G. (2019). Sleepy anger: Restricted sleep amplifies angry feelings. Journal of Experimental Psychology, 148(7), 1239.

Martin, R. C., & Dahlen, E. R. (2005). Cognitive emotion regulation in the prediction of depression, anxiety, stress, and anger. Personality and Individual Differences, 39(7), 1249-1260. doi:10.1016/j.paid.2005.06.004

Monteiro, F., Fonseca, A., Pereira, M., Alves, S., & Canavarro, M. C. (2019). What protects at-risk postpartum women from developing depressive and anxiety symptoms? The role of acceptance-focused processes and self-compassion. Journal of Affective Disorders, 246, 522-529.

Ou, C. H., & Hall, W. A. (2018). Anger in the context of postnatal depression: An integrative review. Birth. Advanced Online Publication. doi.org/10.1111/birt.12356

Potegal, M., Stemmler, G., Spielberger, C. D. (2010). International handbook of anger: Constituent and concomitant biological, psychological, and social processes (1st ed.). New York: Springer.

Simon, R. W., & Lively, K. (2010). Sex, anger and depression. Social Forces, 88(4), 1543-1568.

Tavris, C. (1989). Anger: The misunderstood emotion (Rev. ed.). New York: Simon & Schuster.

Vliegen, N., Casalin, S., Luyten, P., Docx, R., Lenaerts, M., Tang, E., & Kempke, S. (2013). Hospitalization-based treatment for postpartum depressed mothers and their babies: rationale, principles, and preliminary follow-up data. Psychiatry: Interpersonal & Biological Processes, 76(2), 150-168.

THE PAST, PRESENT, AND FUTURE OF PERINATAL MENTAL HEALTH

Brockington I. A historical perspective on the psychiatry of motherhood. In: Riecher-Rossler A, editor. Perinatal Stress, Mood and Anxiety Disorders. Basel: Karger; 2005. p. 1-5.

Coble P.A., Day N.L. (1988) The Epidemiology of Mental and Emotional Disorders during Pregnancy and the Postpartum Period. In: Psychiatric Consultation in Childbirth Settings. Springer, Boston, MA. https://doi.org/10.1007/978-1-4684-5439-0_4

Marks MN. Introduction: Professor Channi Kumar (1938-2000). Br J Psychiatry Suppl. 2004 Feb;46:s1-2. PMID: 14754811.

Pawluski JL, Lonstein JS, Fleming AS. The Neurobiology of Postpartum Anxiety and Depression. Trends Neurosci. 2017;40(2):106-20.

Sharma, V., Santopinto, A. Childbirth and Manic-Depressive Illness: An Account of Emil Kraepelin's Contribution. German J Psychiatry 2008; 11: 168-172).

Trede K, Baldessarini RJ, Viguera AC, Bottero A. Treatise on insanity in pregnant, postpartum, and lactating women (1858) by Louis-Victor Marcé: a commentary. Harv Rev Psychiatry. 2009;17(2):157-65. doi: 10.1080/10673220902891802. PMID: 19373623.

Robert Sparks Essay Context, May 3, 2013. Sadness and Support: A Short History of Postpartum Depression. https://medicine.uiowa.edu/bioethics/bioethics/sites/medicine.uiowa.edu.bioethics/files/wysiwyg_uploads/2013%20Rysavy%20essay.pdf

Made in the USA
Monee, IL
11 January 2022

88705348R00204